TOOLKIT FOR CAREGIVERS

TIPS, SKILLS, AND WISDOM TO MAXIMIZE
YOUR TIME TOGETHER

DEIDRE EDWARDS

ALSO BY THIS AUTHOR

Toolkit for Wellness—Master Your Health and Stress Response for Life

Tired of feeling frustrated about starting new, healthy habits? Do the promises you make to yourself on January 1st become distant reminders of failure by January 15th?

Toolkit for Wellness will shed light on why you are NOT a failure, and will give you the tools for assured success in improved health, reduced stress response—and an actual, doable, habit-changing process that will revolutionize your approach to life itself!

By employing, Deidre's Easy Tweaks Method, you will rock at living an anti-inflammatory life inside and out.

Toolkit for Wellness will enable you to achieve the health you long for through understanding and applying the concepts behind:

- Tweaking Habits
- Maintaining Change Easily
- Nutrient Dense Foods
- Anti-inflammatory Eating
- Great Gut Health
- Quick Workouts at Home

Armed with a new view of how foods are broken down by and react with the body, readers will be able to apply these principles right away for immediate improvements in their health and well-being.

This is your answer to stop that downward-spiraling stress response, starting daily habit 'tweaks' that will revolutionize your life and health, easily exercising at home, and removing the confusion about what is good to eat and why.

BONUS FEATURES OF THIS EDITION

**Welcome to the 2-in-1 Caregiver Combo!
With this purchase you are getting *two* books in one!**

**I just knew my readers would need *both* Toolkits for
all of their caregiving needs!
Toolkit for Caregivers will take you through the daily
tasks, skills, and concerns of caregiving, and *Love
Lives Here: Toolkit for Caregiver Survival* will help
smooth your caregiving path before, during, and even
after your time of being a caregiver is completed.**

**As an extra gift, I am offering a link to FREE,
downloadable, and printable skills sheets. Each skill
that is covered in *Toolkit for Caregivers* will be
available for readers to print out. These skills sheets
can easily be kept within reach while you perform any
basic, yet unfamiliar, caregiving tasks.**

**Simply visit https://deidreedwards.com/index.php/
tk4c-bonus-materials/ to access them.**

CONTENTS

TOOLKIT FOR CAREGIVERS

LOVE LIVES HERE

TOOLKIT FOR CAREGIVERS

TIPS, SKILLS, AND WISDOM TO MAXIMIZE
YOUR TIME TOGETHER

For Virgil, James, and Serena

This book is dedicated to the millions of caregivers who are giving their hearts, bodies, and souls to make sure their loved ones/patients have the best home care possible.

This is also dedicated to my dear husband, Virgil, who supported me through this whole process and was the sweetest patient anyone could ever have.

FOREWORD

We caregivers are not alone. We may feel lost and alone at times—exhausted and overwhelmed, too—and on our last gossamer-thin thread.

Yet, another day dawns and we are needed. Desperately needed by a loved one/patient whose world has shrunk to the size of a bed.

Whether it's by sudden accident, the ravages of an insidious disease, or the cumulative effects of aging, we caregivers—my dear reader—are legion.

A 2015 study by the National Alliance for Caregiving, (NAC), in collaboration with the American Association of Retired Persons, (AARP, Inc.), cited some facts confirming the sweeping effects of the caregiving role.[1]

See if you can't find yourself somewhere in the following points gleaned from that comprehensive study:

- Approximately 34.2 million Americans have been

caregivers for someone 50 years old or older in the last 12 months
- Sixty percent (60%) of those caregivers are female
- Twenty percent (20%) of those caregivers are taking care of more than one person
- The average age of the caregiver is 49 years
- Three out of five care recipients have long-term conditions
- Twenty-five percent (25%) of the care recipients have memory problems
- If the caregiver is a spouse/partner, nearly 45 hours per week will be spent in caregiving activities
- Nearly sixty percent (60%) of the care activity is spent with ADL's—Activities of Daily Living—(bathing, dressing, grooming, feeding, etc.)
- Twenty-five percent (25%) of the caregivers find performing ADL's difficult—especially activities dealing with urination, bowel movements, and bathing
- Six out of ten caregivers perform nursing tasks such as injections, tube feedings, and colostomy care; and many of those feel under-prepared to do those tasks
- One-half of all caregivers had no choice in becoming a caregiver
- The longer a caregiver does the tasks of caregiving, the more likely they will report a decrease in their own health status
- Caregiving for a close relative such as a spouse or parent is reportedly the most emotionally stressful
- Having someone requiring a caregiver creates financial stress

Perhaps the list I just mentioned has ticked off a lot of your own boxes. It certainly did for me. I would highly recommend you read the entire study; but the point is—you are not alone. While I can't promise to provide insight to all your caregiving issues, I hope to help you see how I have addressed many of the common issues that come with having a loved one/patient confined to a hospital bed at home.

_____

1. http://www.caregiving.org/caregiving2015/

DISCLAIMER

This book is the story of how I did the caregiving for my husband. It is not intended to be an official comprehensive training manual for family caregivers or for professionals providing care.

If you received this book through an agency that provides any kind of caregiving or caregiving supplies, the forwarding agency is not responsible for the content or accuracy of the information contained in this book and is not responsible for the outcome of anyone using the techniques or methods described therein.

Also, if you received this book through an agency unaffiliated with health care—religious, civic, profit, or not for profit, etc.—that agency is not responsible for the content or accuracy of the information contained in this book; nor are they responsible for the outcome of anyone using various techniques or methods referred to therein.

Readers should seek the advice of their physician, home health, or Hospice agency before using any ideas or techniques shared from my personal experiences. Individual differences in a patient's and caregiver's own health may change the safety or advisability of using any of the techniques listed or discussed in this book.

I am not responsible for the safety and welfare, or the health status of any patient, health care provider, or caregiver using any of the techniques or information I describe. I am in no way responsible for how any reader interprets or applies this information.

The mention of various products or stores in this book does not constitute my endorsement of said products or businesses. I received no financial compensation from the manufacturers of those products or from the businesses that sell them.

INTRODUCTION

Are you one of the millions of people who has become a caregiver? It is easily one of the most daunting tasks ever given to someone, especially if your loved one/patient is confined to bed.

I know this personally. I've just recently hung up my caregiver wings.

Having been an RN who spent nearly 18 years teaching others how to be Certified Nursing Assistants, or CNAs, I thought I had a handle on what this new role of being a caregiver would entail. I was only partially right. Doing most of the caregiving tasks was not so difficult, thanks to my previous training; but I had practically no experience working with home health and Hospice agencies—nor did I know how they worked. The pathway of adapting my skill set to the home venue was a mystery yet to be discovered and figured out.

Any feelings of emotional stability, regarding my response to our radical change in lifestyle, was a distant wish. I was not prepared for the jumble of grief-related emotions that would overcome me. I taught *others* about the stages of grief, but I didn't want to go through them *myself*. The feelings of guilt blind-sided me as I dared to think about what I was no longer able to do because of the inherent restrictions of being a 24/7 caregiver. Not knowing when or how I would lose my husband haunted me every day.

I can only imagine how you, someone looking for help, answers, or a lifeline, must feel about now:

> Overwhelmed?
> Scared?
> Afraid?
> Unsure?
> Thinking you may not be up to the task?

Help is on the way! With the practical advice and helpful tips contained in this book, you will make your loved one/patient safer, more comfortable, and yes, even happy. You can be spared a lot of trial-and-error, as well as fumbling mistakes because you will already have some "tricks in your bag" to make home care for your bedridden loved one/patient so much easier for both of you.

You will soon learn about the ins-and-outs of the following topics:

- **The physical environment**—From hospital beds at home, bedside commodes, over-the-bed tables and linens —to creating a cheerful, stimulating atmosphere for the patient and you
- **Processes for patient care**—Eating, drinking, urination, bowel movements, positioning, rolling, bathing, shaving, hair and nail care, feeding, and more ...
- **Processes for you the caregiver**—Calendars, getting additional help, tips to save time in the kitchen, taking care of yourself, and ways to cope

- **Processes for home visits**—Making the most of visits from Home Health and Hospice aides, nurses, therapists, social workers, and pastoral care
- **Bringing the party home**—Activities that can stimulate, soothe, and re-energize everyone

Have I mentioned some things you were wondering about—or maybe have never heard of before? That's okay. I've got you covered!

Part of the stress of being a caregiver is feeling like you've entered a maze in a dark room and your task is to successfully navigate to the other side with no instructions and no flash light.

There is a better way!

My sincere desire is to help you along the way, turning on the lights and giving you a map that will assist you in taking some of that caregiving burden off your shoulders.

Granted, each situation is unique. There is no *average* bedridden or Hospice patient. Every home environment and family dynamic are different. I just know, even with my medical background, I would have loved to have had **someone** to give me this book full of tips and ideas, so I could have had more confidence and practical know-how *from the start*.

What I *can* do, is hand this book to you!

You're welcome!

Now, let's get started.

1

PHYSICAL ENVIRONMENT

One immediate concern for us caregivers is what to do with all the medical equipment that soon becomes a daily presence in our world. This chapter takes you through the basic equipment, supplies, and concerns that can easily overwhelm your household and unravel your nerves with endless learning curves.

Relax.

I will explain it all right here starting with the bedroom and take you through making the home hospital bed more comfortable for the patient and user-friendly for caregivers. I will familiarize you with other equipment that may be needed along with tips on how to use it. You will also be introduced to the daily supplies for patient care and how they are used for maximum benefit.

Let's start shining a bright light onto the unfamiliar world of medical equipment so you can begin to feel more confident right away.

The Bedroom—Where to put the home hospital bed and over-bed table

The addition of a hospital bed to your home should be a blessed relief. Safely caring for someone who is totally—or mostly—bedridden at home is exhausting using a regular bed. Sore backs, along with the stress and strain of bending over a domestic bed are over. Hallelujah!

Care must be taken when choosing where to put the bed. Here is a list of the many factors to consider:

- Space available
- Accessibility to both sides of the bed
- Privacy
- The fact your patient's world will be pretty much confined to this space
- If you want to sleep in the same room as your loved one/patient

Your response to the above factors may change over time but be mindful that relocating the hospital bed in a home is not easily done. Unlike hospitals with linoleum floors and wide doorways, homes are usually not set up to roll beds from room to room.

Other equipment you will need for someone who is mostly or partially confined to bed is an over-the-bed table. This item was not covered by our insurance, but having one is essential for eating, keeping personal items close by, and for the caregiving processes.

We bought ours outright, but you can check with second-hand stores, friends, and your home health care organization or Hospice agency for the availability of used over-the-bed tables.

Protect Your Floors

Keep in mind all life and bodily functions are going to happen in this space. Where are the drips and crumbs going to fall? Where will the bath water splash? How about drops of urine? Imagine how your floors might look after a urine or food spill disaster!

We had just installed brand new plush wall-to-wall carpeting throughout our house when my husband became bedridden. Yikes! Even if we had hardwood flooring, there was no way I was going to damage the floors with the inevitable spills that happen.

Enter carpet protectors from the local office supply store. I purchased the largest one they had for the "business" side of the bed, (over-the-bed table side), and a smaller one for the other side where the urinary drainage bag would hang. These are the protectors designed for office desk chairs to roll about on but work wonders for easy maneuvering of the over-the-bed table and catching a multitude of drips and crumbs from eating, drinking, and personal care.

Something to Look At

There is no telling how long your loved one/patient may live in this room. Think about it.

Live. In. This. Room.

The prevailing thought at the time of my husband's being placed into Hospice care, was that he'd have only a few months to live. In fact, he spent over two years confined to bed and under Hospice's and my care!

No matter how long your bedridden loved one/patient lives in that bed and space, that is their WORLD.

Make their world as pleasant to their senses as possible.

Are there windows to look out of from their vantage point? More than any other direction, they will be looking straight ahead.

Is there a window view in this direction? If not, make sure the wall they are facing is beautiful! While family pictures should be around, I found my husband getting "lost" in the beautiful landscape picture that hung in his direct view. We even rotated landscape pictures with the seasons.

A calendar, especially a 'Today Is ' variety, is handy for reality orientation. A clock that is easy to read is a real plus, too.

I will address other ways to dress up your loved one/patient's space in the *Bring the Party Home* chapter.

The Bed Itself—Size Matters

If your loved one/patient is tall—say six feet or over—you should discuss the options with the equipment providers. Quite possibly, you may need a bed extension. I was unaware of this possibility and we had to put up with a shorter bed for months before we went through the hassle of changing out my husband's bed. Save your loved one/patient the process of being suspended in a Hoyer lift for 10-15 minutes while the bed is being switched out by FIRST discussing the availability of a longer bed BEFORE they start living in it.

Slip 'N Slide

Bed length matters because of the mysterious process of daily *patient drift*—the mechanics and dynamics of going back and forth from a lying down position to a sitting up position several times a day, create a 'slip 'n slide' effect resulting in the patient slipping down toward the foot of the bed.

Tall patients end up *standing* in bed very quickly, even though they may be lying high up on the mattress at the start of the day. Shorter patients still drift to the foot of the bed; but they have a bigger margin of error before their feet get jammed into the footboards. Even so, a shorter patient will end up bending more in their chest area than at their waist if not properly pulled up in bed.

There can also be a side-to-side drift.

How we assist in moving patients up in bed will be discussed in the *Processes for the Patient* chapter.

Electric vs. Manual

Standard-issue home hospital beds in our area are electrically controlled. Yay! But power failures do happen. Before the bed installer leaves, make sure you know where the crank is and how to operate it. Better yet, have the installer take the crank out from where it is hiding, generally somewhere between the mattress and the box springs, and do a demonstration on how to use it.

Afterwards, keep the crank on the floor and/or under the bed for easy emergency access. Nothing like fumbling in the dark for the crank in the middle of a power outage and raging storm.

The Height of a Bed

One of the wonders of hospital-type beds is the fact they can be raised to a good working height for the care provider. No more bending over a low bed to give patient care.

One of the first things medical people learn is to always leave the room with the patient bed in its lowest position with the side rails raised. Why? You do not want the patient to fall out of bed—especially from great heights.

If your loved one/patient is of sound mind, this rule may be bent at home if you so choose and the doctor agrees. I was in and out of my husband's room all the time. If he was awake, we hugged just about every time I came into his room. Keeping his bed elevated just made sense for us.

If he had lost his faculties and tried to get out of bed, then I would have kept his bed down in its lowest position and just raised it up each time for his care.

This vital safety issue needs to be further discussed with your home healthcare provider or Hospice agency.

A Bed of Many Layers

Home hospital bed mattresses are not soft. While a firm foundation is a good thing, bedridden folks need constant protection from the ravages of bed sores, pressure sores, decubitus ulcers ... whatever you want to call them.

Bed Sores vs. Kennedy Ulcers

If a caregiver's loved one/patient develops any kind of bed sore, there's often an overwhelming sense of guilt. Bed sores, pressure ulcers, or decubitus ulcers are often seen as a sign of poor patient care because they can often be avoided through good nutrition, regularly changing body positions every two hours, and good hygiene.

Guilt is usually neither helpful nor productive. Quite possibly, understanding the bigger picture for the patient, and yourself, will create a better outcome for you both. Chances are, you are not letting your loved one/patient lie in bed with a soiled, wet brief for hours. If your loved one/patient is in Hospice care, what you may be seeing is a Kennedy Ulcer.

Called Kennedy Terminal Ulcers, this form of skin breakdown— often in the sacral area of the buttocks—is a sign of further body deterioration and body system failure. It is yet another box that is often ticked off as the terminal patient's condition declines.

While I have seen pressure sores, which were left unchecked, eat away at the flesh all the way to the bone, the Kennedy Ulcer I saw in my husband never progressed from its fairly superficial skin layer involvement. The sacral area of the buttocks may appear deeply black-and-blue and very unhappy (red and irritated). The very delicate outer layer of skin that regenerates will easily slough off even with gentle cleansing.

What worked for us was the combo barrier cream described later in this book, no dressings applied, and a lot of TLC, when moving him in bed and during bathing.

More About Bed Layers

To help with skin breakdown issues from lying in bed 24/7, ask your doctor for an alternating air pressure mattress—by prescription. This lovely device fills and releases channels of air underneath the patient to change pressure points. It goes on top of the mattress provided. The motor that runs this should be virtually silent. If the motor is noisy, ask for a newer model. We endured a noisy motor for months not knowing there was a better option.

But an alternating air pressure mattress itself is not soft or cushy either. Enter the memory foam layer! This is the heavenly layer that provides the "ahhh" moment and the cuddly "cush" your loved one/patient deserves. You may have to purchase this yourself. It is readily available in most stores or online. Twin size works for most.

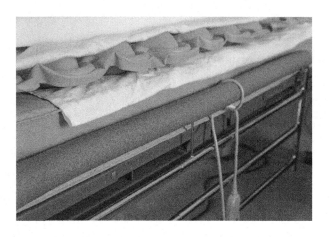

Pool Noodles?

Using pool noodles to cover the bed rails has been the best trick ever. This one idea is just golden.

Aside from looking so ... sterile ... so ... medical, home hospital beds are SO COLD TO TOUCH. The metal side rails, so important for patient safety and for turning, are hard, cold, and downright unfriendly to even bump into.

Let me introduce the colorful, temperature-neutral, and cushioning pool noodle!

Simply slice through one side of the small-sized pool noodle lengthwise to open it up. Press the cut opening of the noodle over the top of the bedside rails. You can trim the length to fit, but we didn't find it necessary. Some patients thrash around a bit, and these pool noodles can save a few bruises. At all times, they create a nice surface for both the patient and anyone attending him/her to lean their arms or hands on.

We used a medium-sized pool noodle to fit over the top of the footboard. This one we trimmed to fit.

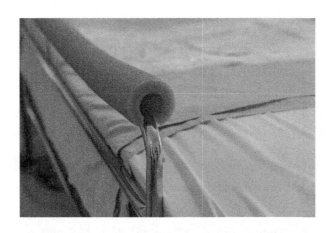

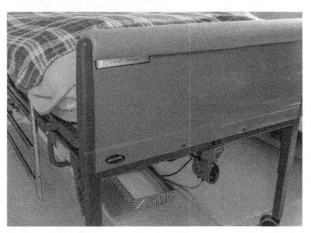

Pool noodles to the rescue again. One very important element to skin care!

A very important factor in maintaining skin care and avoiding pressure points is protecting the patient's feet from being rubbed by the covers and blankets. You can easily triumph over this by placing two shorter lengths of small pool noodles to stand up at the end of the bed (like goal posts) and using the bed frame to hold them. All sheets and blankets can be draped over these to create a "no touch zone" for the feet.

If there are ulcerative, burned, or other skin care concerns farther up the body, one or two full length pool noodles can easily be bent over the patient's legs, so no covers will touch the lower extremities. The noodles are simply pushed between the side of the mattress and the side rails.

Yet another use for pool noodles, we discovered, was to place the length of the jumbo-sized noodle to fit between the end of the mattress and the footboard. The larger noodle helps to prevent the mattress from sliding down to the footboard. The jumbo size was, actually, not 'fat' enough to do the job, so I rolled a bath towel around it to make a tighter fit.

Success again!

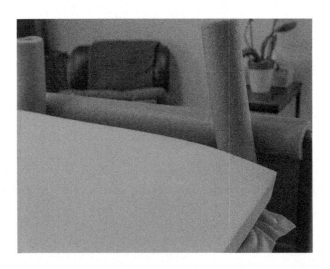

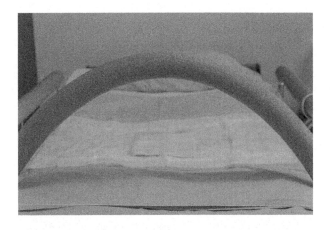

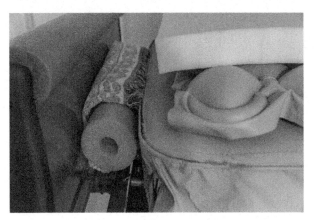

Draw Sheets

Draw sheets provide many advantages and are where the magic happens!

- Draw sheets allow one person to turn even a large patient alone.
- Draw sheets allow two people to "oop" the patient from side-to-side or up in the bed.
- Draw sheets protect the fitted sheet and all the layers below.

- Draw sheets can be easily changed rather than having a total change of linens.

So, what are draw sheets?

At home, draw sheets can be created from any-sized flat sheet. For the main draw sheet under my husband, I used flat queen-sized sheets. Fold the flat sheet so top and bottom hems meet. You now have a sheet folded in half, with a side that has a fold and a side that is open, with the two hems on top of each other. Bring the corners of the folded side together. Now you have a sheet folded into quarters. Place the side edge that is folded over the others across the bed (on top of the fitted sheet) in line with where the patient's shoulders would go.

Diagram showing how to fold a queen size flat sheet to create a draw sheet

 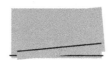

Note the top and bottom hems of the open flat sheet. Make the first fold by putting the hem ends together. Make sure there are no wrinkles and the hems meet square at the bottom.

You now have one fold and the hem ends are together.

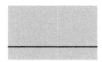

Bring the folded corners of the sheet together to create the last fold. You now have a sheet folded into quarters. Make sure all layers are smooth.

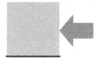

The fold on the side (arrow) will be placed horizontally across the top of the bed in line with the patients's shoulders.

Make sure all layers are smooth. With the final fold placed at the top of the bed, there will less of a tendency to wrinkle as the patient moves.

Smooth the rest of this folded sheet down the bed. NO WRINKLES! Wrinkles cause skin problems. The folded flat sheet should extend from the shoulder area through to the upper thigh area of the patient.

If you have added the additional layers I have recommended, (alternating air pressure mattress and memory foam), I suggest **additional draw sheets**—one under the memory foam and another one under the air mattress. These draw sheets can be of simpler form and not folded into quarters. They could be a twin flat sheet folded once so the hems meet. Align these simpler draw sheets the same way under the patient as with the regular draw sheet—meaning extending from the patient's shoulder area to thigh area.

Diagram of the patient bed layers we used, from bottom-up:

Mattress (black)
Single-layer (unfolded) draw sheet (white)
Alternating air pressure mattress (gray)
Single-layer draw sheet (white)
Two-inch memory foam mattress topper (off white)

The bed linens go directly on top of the memory foam.
The fitted sheet should cover all layers shown below (get deep pockets).

Not only do patients magically drift around the bed, but the different layers drift as well. These additional draw sheets will enable you and one other person to have near pinpoint accuracy in rearranging the different layers of the bed.

Because these additional draw sheets hang off the bed sides, simply tuck them under the mattress to neaten them up. The fitted sheet covers up everything.

Blue-backed absorbent pads

Another friend to the bedridden patient and the caregivers is the absorbent and disposable blue pad. They absorb moisture of all kinds while keeping the draw sheet and the under-lying fitted sheet dry.

Adult briefs can leak body fluids; and catheters can leak urine due to bladder spasms. Even if your patient is continent (in control of) his/her bowels, an episode of "gas" can cause unintentional leakage of bowel movement (BM).

To avoid various degrees of bed linen changes, the blue pad can do the job and is easily replaced. The home healthcare representative or Hospice aide can show you how to do this, but it will require two rolling processes for the patient—once to the right and once to the left.

If the patient is not wearing an adult brief, a mini blue pad may be added to catch "dirty gas" and not require extensive movement.

Let me explain:

- Blue pads are placed, blue side DOWN, under the patient's buttocks.
- Whole blue pads may be cut into 8 pieces each (see picture) and can be accurately placed while the patient is on one side. The goal is to place the small pad to cover the anus and extend down and away from the anus.

Diagram of Patient in bed, showing fitted sheet (medium gray), folded draw sheet (light gray) and blue pad (dark gray)

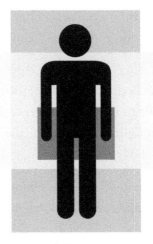

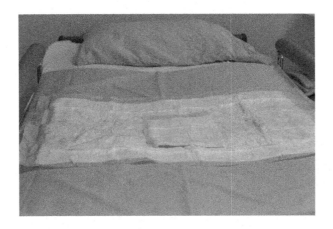

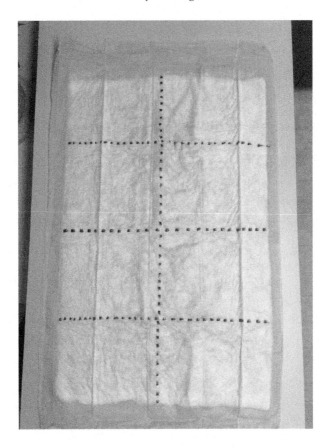

Linens

After well over two years, we were still going strong on just two sets of twin-sized sheets, two bed draw sheets, and a couple extra pillows with cases for positioning. A single micro-plush blanket is adequate for daily warmth.

At night, I added a super-soft, feather-light, cuddly lap blanket folded double for the shoulder and upper-chest area. In the colder months, I used a very light down-type throw over the whole bed.

It can be easy to over-heat the patient, which can cause heat rash issues on the back, upper thigh/groin areas, or anywhere there are skin folds. Keep an eye on the skin to judge how much warmth is tolerated.

Crumb Catchers—NOT Bibs

Using the same thinking that implies adults use briefs and not diapers, we use crumb catchers and not bibs. Hospitals often call these clothing protectors, but that sounds a little sterile to me. We could always get a laugh or start a fun conversation when referring to the crumb catcher saving a bite of oatmeal spontaneously taking a plunge off the spoon!

Crumb catchers can simply consist of a hand towel tucked around the neckline and running lengthwise down the patient's chest. If you are handy with a sewing machine, cutting a hand towel to fit around the neck, and creating Velcro or tie attachments, is not difficult. We acquired a finished one from a brief Hospice facility stay that was sent home with him—so we used the "fancy" one and the occasional hand towel to "catch" those crumbs trying to escape!

Rub-a-dub-dub

Washcloths and more washcloths. We went through more washcloths than anything else. Did I say we used a lot of washcloths?

Who knew there are so many levels of quality and thickness to washcloths? The ones in hospitals and nursing homes are purchased by the gross and can often be kissing cousins to sandpaper. The other extreme might be found in a luxury hotel where the ever-so-plush washcloth could not dry out overnight if its life depended on it.

Caregiving requires washcloths that have a degree of softness but that can also dry out in a reasonable amount of time. Most of us are aware, a wet washcloth will sour quickly. I have tried all sorts of home and manufactured products to redeem a soured washcloth or towel and have failed miserably. Living in the humid South, we must be very careful about souring of the towels, anyway.

I have been most satisfied with the eight-pack washcloths that Target offers. At any time, I had three or four of their washcloth packs in multiple colors all washed and folded to be used exclusively for patient care. When the yellow ones, for example, began to get stained or became scratchy, I easily pulled that set and grabbed some more from the linen closet. For ease of use, keep these accessible in the nearest bathroom to the patient where caregiving supplies are kept.

Why so many washcloths?

First, for sanitation reasons, they should be used once and then laundered. If you are not doing a load of laundry that day, hang the squeezed-out washcloths on a towel rod or drape them over the edge of the laundry room sink so they can dry out.

Second, during bed baths, using a washcloth to **dry,** as well as wash, is so much easier. The bath towel is used mostly to cover the patient for warmth and modesty. Rather than flapping and dragging around a big towel to dry the patient, simply grabbing another washcloth to dry is more user-friendly to both the caregiver and the patient. That's another reason for multiple colors ... the blue one today is for washing ... the green one is for drying, etc.

Pre-Moistened Wipes vs. Toilet Tissue

Someone who has compromised health and is largely lying in bed all day is going to have skin issues—especially around the buttocks. Wiping bottoms with toilet tissue can tear up the skin—as can a washcloth.

To avoid abrading this delicate and challenged area, pre-moistened wipes are a wonder! I learned a trick from one of our Hospice aides to tear the cloths in half. When completely unfolded, the brand we were given by Hospice had long moist sheets. You can get so much more mileage out of one wipe if you first tear it into two pieces.

Also, if room temperature wipes are too cold, they can easily be dipped into a pan of warm water first. There are also devices that warm pre-moistened wipes, which can be purchased in the baby supply departments of some stores and can possibly save you a step or two.

Butt Paste

Butt Paste or Butt Cream are rather indelicate terms for a vital product often called a barrier cream. We have used three different kinds based on the needs of the skin.

Being bedridden places an enormous strain on the integrity of the buttocks and other pressure points. That's why we had several added layers to my husband's hospital bed. That's also why Butt Paste/Cream needs to be applied to the entire buttocks "sitting" area after each cleaning. These creams can also be applied to elbows and heels—anywhere showing wear and tear.

Consult with your home health or Hospice nurse on which kind you should use.

Barrier Cream Combo

After much trial and error, a Hospice nurse recommended we combine a product called Aloe Vesta Protective Ointment with another cream that was very thick, pink, and contained zinc and calamine. Once we landed on this combination for the "butt cream," we were able to stabilize my husband's areas of concern.

At one time, we had even used thick 7-day protective wound patches, but even they seemed to irritate the areas around the edge of the spot we were trying to protect. Truly, for us, this combo cream was miraculous—as my husband laid on his backside all day long.

I just used a clean, empty face cream type of jar, squeezed some of each cream into it, and stirred the concoction with my gloved finger. It's a cinch. Another of our Hospice nurses went to Dollar Tree just to buy jars for her patients to use so they could do the same thing. Hospice nurses are wonderful!

But Wait—There's More!

There is an issue about pink barrier cream, however, even when used in the combo cream described above.

It. Will. Not. Wipe. Off.

As tempting as it might be to give up and just keep layering the cream on, it is important to take the affected area down to zero at least once a day. Skin assessment is paramount; and it can't be done through a layer of pink cream.

I discovered a solution. When normal body wash was not doing the job at all, we were stymied. We couldn't use Ajax and a scrub brush —this was delicate skin. I turned to a product I use on my face that is super gentle and yet effectively removes make up—mascara included.

Enter Cetaphil Daily Facial Cleanser. It just takes a couple of squirts of Cetaphil on a gloved hand and a gentle circular rubbing of the affected area—the pink residue can be wiped off using a pre-moistened disposable towelette. Magic!

Body Creams or lotions?

I have found that body creams are much more effective for moisturizing than lotions. In fact, I augment my own hand/body cream with a small amount of coconut oil. Our nurses and aides raved about this mixture, and I know it worked well—not only on my husband, but for me!

I start with a jar of Cetaphil Moisturizing Cream and stir in 2-3 tablespoons of coconut oil. This non-greasy combination will do wonders for dried skin, keeping it hydrated and smooth.

Bedside Commodes

If your loved one/patient is still weight bearing and can tolerate being upright, a bedside commode can be so handy in order to maintain some resemblance of normality and dignity for bathroom processes.

Having said that, it can in some ways create more work for the caregiver and can ramp up safety concerns.

Let me explain.

- There's the transfer. Your home health worker or Hospice agency can show you how to safely transfer your loved one/patient from the bed to the bedside commode. It takes strength and balance on the caregiver's part. Seriously ill patients are subject to getting lightheaded while being upright, and caregivers need to be "on the ready" for a safe, rapid return of the patient to a lying down position.

- Bedside commodes need to be emptied. Urine and bowel movements must be transferred to the bathroom toilet as soon as possible—lest the patient environment starts smelling quite bad. Pouring out urine into the toilet and rinsing the pan is relatively easy. Transferring BM's is problematic and much more hands-on—gloved, of course.

We went through the bedside commode phase until it was no longer a safe choice. Catheters have their own issues, too; but when safely exiting the bed was no longer a possibility and changing wet adult briefs was almost impossible, the cleanliness and convenience of a catheter won out.

Speaking of Catheters...

The longer a patient has an indwelling urinary catheter, the greater chance there is for a bladder infection. At the same time, a catheter will eliminate caustic urine from irritating or breaking down skin. It's a choice you must discuss with your doctor and nurse.

Catheters are changed out, as a rule, every 30 days. Your home health provider or Hospice nurse will do this. There are sometimes extenuating medical circumstances that might modify that schedule.

You may want to request an adhesive leg stabilizer for the catheter tubing rather than the customary leg strap. We found the elastic leg strap to be more of a bother. The adhesive product has a snap-on center for the tubing that rotates easily for changing which side of the bed the bag is hanging on.

Purple Bag Syndrome? Yup. The urinary drainage bag (especially) and the tubing can become discolored and turn a purple-blue. Relax! It's not the end of the world. For whatever reason, the patient's urine's chemical composition reacts with the bag and tubing. This urine may also have a stronger scent.

Okay. It stinks.

Fortunately, the external tubing and the bag can be changed out more frequently. The nurse can do this every week if it becomes a problem.

Room Deodorizers

Life can get stinky—but the heavy smell of room sprays can be suffocating to sensitive noses or simply smell like a cover-up to poor care.

For the naturalists and pure-minded, an open box lid filled with baking soda placed under the hospital bed may do the trick.

Different wound infections, or Purple Bag Syndrome situations, may require something stronger. A jar of odor-removing gel beads should freshen up the scent. When new, these jars may seem strong smelling. In that case, cover part of the open lattice lid with plastic wrap. Eventually, these gel beads disappear and you'll need a new jar.

For bowel movements, a lit candle can eliminate odors in a few minutes. However, if there's any chance someone could knock it over or forget about it, this may present a safety issue. If that is the concern, an open window may be your best choice.

Hoyer Lifts

Hoyer is actually a brand name but has become a universal term for mechanical lifts. Whatever you call them, they are a blessing. They can also become a deadly curse when operated by novices or without enough extra help.

A mechanical lift can get the bedridden patient totally airborne with no body part touching the bed. They are, however, so scary to be in. Much reassurance needs to be given to the patient, and plenty of hands need to be available to help hold dangling legs or to support the patient's head.

Wow! Why even use these scary things? These mechanical lifts can help transfer a non-ambulatory and non-weight bearing patient to a wheelchair or recliner. We used the Hoyer lift to simply raise my husband off the bed enough for us to rearrange and straighten the bed layers, when no amount of using draw sheets could realign things.

If you have room to store one, even a once-a-month use by capable hands can justify having one. Talk to your home health provider or Hospice agency about the advisability of getting a mechanical lift. You also need to have a firm understanding about who can operate it and how they are trained.

My own personal rule was to have no fewer than three people present for mechanical lift use for my husband who could not readily move or control his legs. Even with less handicapped patients, there should always be two people present—in my opinion.

So Much Trash!

The patient care area needs its own trash system. I recycled the grocery store plastic bags that so easily accumulate and use the white ones in the patient care area because they looked clean. Hey, I'm a nurse. This bag easily hung on the closet door handle near the bed.

From used tissues, supply packaging, used Clorox wipes to poo-stained blue pads, and BM itself, these bags are so useful and can easily be tied off and placed in the garbage can.

If your state has outlawed plastic store bags, I would recommend purchasing some small white trashcan liners. These bags easily fill up during the course of a day and you want to remove any source of bad smells right away.

Can You Hear Me Now?

Hospitals and nursing homes have call bell systems. At home we have... what?

A cow bell? Might be hard to use and it could wake up the neighbors.

Voice? "I called you and called you! Where were you?" You were probably in deep REM sleep.

Walkie-Talkie? There are 28 channels to choose from; some require you to apply to the FCC... Okay, we used channel 1- but so did the hunters at the break of dawn. So did some ladies traveling down the interstate. You see, these devices have a range of 10 miles. Oh, and they need to be charged for 16 hours every day.

Forget it.

Enter the customer service bell! Ding! I was usually on my feet after the first clang but even just a few of those would wake me from deep sleep ... and I often slept on the other side of the house.

Where are you?

Suppose your loved one/patient has been sleeping for hours and you want to step outside for a few minutes? One way is to create signs that can be left in plain sight on the over-the-bed table.

One day, I neglected to do this. I had just stepped out onto the porch for a few minutes of fresh air. My husband woke up ahead of when I thought he would and was simply terrified at not knowing where I was. He called and called. I couldn't hear him and had not left a note. Talk about feeling regretful and guilt-ridden.

Always leave a note if your loved one/patient is sighted and can read—even if you've only gone out to the porch for a breath of fresh air.

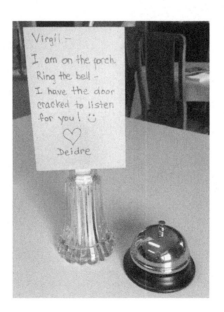

Lessons from Chapter 1

Just knowing in advance about the caregiving concerns dealing with the physical environment, equipment, and medical supplies should help you avoid many pitfalls. Even if you still have any unanswered questions, you will at least have a basis to pose an informed question to your home health or Hospice agency.

Smoothly managing the physical environment will save you so much heartache down the road.

Now that you have mastered the basics of the bed, over-bed table, linens, bathing supplies, body and barrier creams, mechanical lifts, trash, and communication tools, I will help you conquer the world of infection control. You will learn how to easily protect yourself and your loved one/patient from getting or passing on nasty germs.

Don't skip this next chapter. The life you save may be your own!

2

INFECTION CONTROL

This could easily be the most important chapter of all. Don't skip this one just because it is short! Protecting yourself and your loved one/patient from infection is of paramount importance. Whether you are a caregiver for one day, one week, or longer, these rules and guidelines are for YOU. Using the techniques I have outlined for you, infection control will soon be under your mastery.

Gloves

"If it's wet, or used to be wet—and it's not yours, don't touch it without gloves!"

That was the sage advice of one of my nursing instructors. It is the perfect way to describe the scope of preventing the spread of disease. In the medical field, this approach is called Standard or Universal Precautions.

Disease transmission is a two-way street. We usually are most concerned about not getting whatever infection the patient may have. Being mindful of the reverse is just as important. A patient does not need to acquire any infection those around him/her may have.

Because we usually can't always see the presence of disease-causing germs, and because infection can develop suddenly, Standard Precautions dictates that we have to assume that every single body secretion is potentially infected.

We do not choose *when* to use protection; **we use protection all of the time!!**

In the home environment, Standard Precautions is most often seen in the common sense use of gloves when providing personal care, and in the thorough washing of the caregiver's hands after glove removal and disposal.

If you are washing or bathing the patient, shaving, removing/applying dressings, assisting with urination or bowel movements, cleaning/trimming nails, or participating in any other type of hands-on-the-patient care, gloves should be worn. Gloves prevent your hands from coming into contact with your loved one/patient's body secretions including blood, drainage from wounds, semen, vaginal secretions, urine, and bowel movements.

Additionally, gloves should be changed after completing one "dirty" task and going on to another. For example: After you have cleaned an infected toe, change gloves before going to another body area to prevent spreading the toe infection. Even in changing a dressing, new clean gloves should be worn to apply the fresh dressing.

Gloves should be free from any obvious holes. If a hole should appear in your gloves, take them off and get new ones.

Removing Gloves

To remove gloves, use one gloved hand to pinch the area just above the wrist area of the other gloved hand. Gently pull the first glove off—making it inside out. Hold the first removed glove in your remaining gloved hand. Slip an ungloved finger under the cuff of the remaining glove and pull off. The second glove will also be inside out and will contain the first glove inside. Immediately drop the used gloves into the trash and then wash your hands.

———

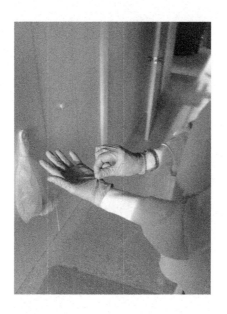

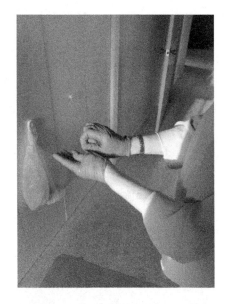

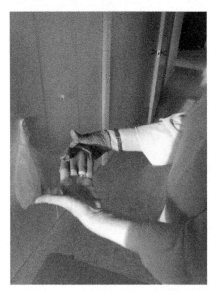

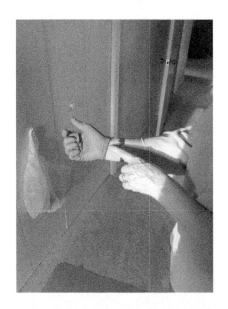

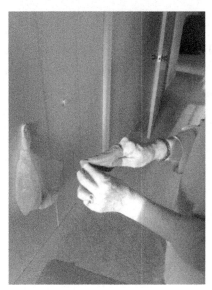

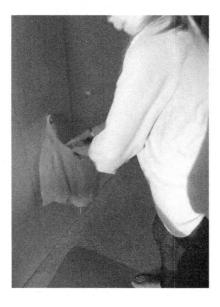

Let me repeat myself. This is VERY important to both of you!

Ask your home health representative or Hospice nurse to show you how to properly apply Standard or Universal Precautions to your loved one/patient's unique situation. In addition to gloves, there are disposable gowns, and masks that can be used to protect caregivers and patients.

Handwashing

We all think we know how to wash our hands. In a caregiving environment, extra attention needs to be given to hand washing techniques. Here are the steps:

———

Hand Washing

- Turn the water on to a comfortably warm temperature and wet your hands
- Apply a squirt of hand soap into your palm
- Hum the "Happy Birthday" song at a normal tempo two times through during the washing phase, which should translate to 20 seconds total. During that time you should:
- Rub the palms together, creating a good lather
- Continue rubbing, moving to the back side of the hands, around the wrist, and between your fingers
- Scrape your fingertips along the palm of the opposite hand, driving the suds under your nails. Repeat for the other hand.
- You should have finished humming "Happy Birthday" twice by now
- Rinse hands under the running water while continuing to rub all areas of the hands, wrist, fingers
- Dry with a clean paper towel.
- Turn off the faucet with a dry paper towel to prevent contamination of your clean hands

————

Lessons from Chapter 2

The bare bones of preventing the spread of infection is through diligent hand washing technique and through the proper use and disposal of gloves. These are the hard and fast rules that apply to anyone taking care of anyone else.

Before you move on, make sure you practice hand washing and putting on and taking off disposable gloves exactly as I have outlined.

. . .

NOTE:

Each of the skills I share with you is also available in a printable PDF form for FREE. Just visit https://deidreedwards.com/index.php/tk4c-bonus-materials/ to easily download and print off each of the skills you want to have at your fingertips. You may want to have them laminated or you can just insert each skill into a plastic binder sleeve to keep in a handy location. If you are learning these things for the first time, having the printed skill to refer to in the patient care area should give you an added layer of security and help boost your confidence.

3

PROCESSES FOR PATIENT CARE

If you are among the millions of caregivers who are over-whelmed by the daily tasks of actually giving care, this chapter was written for you. This is where you will learn the little secrets that will make your caregiving life much easier to handle.

As you learn how to smoothly perform these essential patient care tasks, your confidence will sky-rocket and your loved one/patient will be made so much more comfortable.

We will begin with the basic mechanics of moving a patient up/down or to the right/left of the mattress. Based on how a home hospital bed can be modified for patient comfort found in the first chapter, you will learn how to use those modifications to your and the patient's advantage.

With the ADLs (Activities of Daily Living) covered, you will be able to smoothly bathe, change, shampoo, shave and, generally, give care to the human body. Issues related to eating, drinking, and feeding someone will also be covered to assure the safety and well-being of all concerned.

Let's get started with how to change the patient's position in bed.

Using draw sheets to move the patient in bed

———

Two person technique for moving a patient in bed

- Make sure both caregivers and the patient know what is going to happen before the lift takes place. Start with the bed at a good working height for those doing the move and make sure the bed is fully flat.
- Standing on either side of the patient's bed, two people roll up the edges of the draw sheet until their hands are gripping the rolled sheet near the patient's shoulders and hips
- Using an audible count of "1-2-3" they lift and move the patient right after "3" toward the intended direction of the move (up/down the bed or to the right/left of the bed)
- If the patient is heavier than the two people can safely or successfully move, more people may be used. I have seen four or six people used to lift a patient. Just remember, the goal is not to get the patient airborne as in flipping flapjacks, but to get enough lift to "oop" the patient to a different location in the bed

If you are by yourself and the patient needs to roll to one side or the other for positioning or patient care, draw sheets are invaluable. The following steps will guide you through this process with ease.

———

Rolling a patient to the side using a draw sheet by yourself

- Stand on the side of the bed you want the patient to roll toward.
- Remove top blanket, keeping the top sheet in place.
- If the patient has a catheter, make sure the urinary drainage bag is hanging on the side of the bed where you are standing.
- Pull the top sheet up from the bottom to expose the lower legs.
- Gently scoop up the far leg (under-handed scoop, not an over-handed grip) and cross the far leg over the near leg. A pillow may need to be placed between lower legs, depending on the patient's delicacy.
- Place or instruct the patient to put their hand nearest you to the top of his/her head.
- Place the far hand across the patient's chest or instruct the patient to reach across for the bedrail near you (in the direction of the turn).
- With the patient's arms and legs in place, reach across the patient to grip the far edge of the draw sheet and pull it towards yourself.

———

Voila! The patient will need to hang an arm over the side rail, but since you have padded it with a pool noodle, this is relatively comfortable.

This may sound like a complicated multi-step procedure, but after a time or two, you'll be able to do this in a snap!

Be aware that the patient's ankles may be touching the side rail frame and will, most likely, need cushioning with a pillow or towel to prevent becoming "dented" by the side rail part that is not noodled.

Pointers for moving a patient up in bed by yourself when the patient can't help:

I tried to have someone pass through the house each day to help me move my beloved up in bed. Virtually anyone can help you—more than one friendly visitor had helped me do this. There are times, however, that the patient has migrated to the end of the bed and something must be done—even if you are alone.

This takes great strength, but I successfully moved my 6'2" husband by myself many times.

Here's how:

————

Moving a patient up in bed by yourself

- Make sure the bed is at a good working height for you so you do not have to bend over.
- Lower the head of the bed to the flat position.
- Raise the foot/lower leg section to the highest position.
- Remove the head pillow to cushion the headboard in case you go too far!
- Stand at the head of the bed and roll up the draw sheet corner nearest you, as close to the patient's shoulder as possible. The patient should reach across his chest with his arm nearest to you, if possible.
- Keep the patient informed of your actions and do an audible count before you pull the draw sheet with all your might toward you and the head of the bed. You may need

to do this multiple times. If you are a strength training star or your patient is a "tiny bird," you may not have to pull with such force. No holes in the wall, please!

- Go around to the other side of the bed and repeat.
- Make sure the draw sheet is smooth under the patient.
- Reposition the pillow.
- Lower the foot area of the bed.
- Raise the head of the bed as needed.

————

By raising the foot of the bed, you are enlisting the aid of gravity to help slide the patient toward the head of the bed when you pull on the draw sheet.

Beyond the Commode … How to Handle Poo

Believe me, they never taught us this in nursing school!

Bathrooms. Bedside commodes. Bed pans. Briefs. That's it.

Nobody. Ever. Told. Us. How to help a patient "poo" without using those darned, awful bedpans.

And it's so easy!

If your patient is aware of the need to have a bowel movement, and if transferring to a bedside commode is not a possibility, then there is no reason for them to suffer the indignity of "doing it" in their brief.

Briefs can compound the cleanup process by smooshing the BM all over the patient's private areas. Why have both of you face that clean-up process when you can control where things go?

Here's the secret:

Assisting a bedridden patient with a bowel movement

- Roll the patient to his/her left side (preferably), making sure to cushion the lower legs so they don't bump into the side rails.
- If you are using that mini-blue absorbent pad as previously described, chances are it has caught any early BM. You can augment this "landing zone" by placing 2-3 individual sections of "size-it-yourself" paper towels, right on top of the mini-blue pad, pushing just a bit of the paper towel layer under the buttocks.
- As the BM comes out, you can peel off a layer of paper towel to ready the landing zone for another deposit. **You are, of course, wearing gloves!**
- If this is a formed BM, then you may dump it into the toilet to flush (but not the paper towel) or just put it into a plastic trash bag along with the paper towel.
- As previously described, I recycled plastic grocery store bags. After turning my husband to his side and getting the paper towels in place, I would busy myself with putting the trash bag on the bed (ready for deposits); get a new mini-blue pad ready to put into place post clean up; get the pack of pre-moistened washcloth wipes that Hospice provided and get the tube of Butt Paste or jar of Combo Cream.
- With any luck, all you need to change out is the mini-blue pad.
- Make sure during clean-up to take at least one swipe with a clean half of the pre-moistened wipe up along the bottom buttocks cheek touching the bed. This ensures

that you have not missed cleaning some BM that has hidden out of sight.

- Once everything is done, cleaned up, and creamed, you can remove your gloves, tie off the trash bag, and reposition your patient.
- Now go wash your hands!

————

While nothing can substitute what we have done our entire lives— going to the bathroom and sitting on the commode—this is the easiest way I have found to keep the patient clean and still maintain some level of dignity.

A note for heart failure patients:

At some point in the decline of heart failure patients, rolling to the left side can become problematic for their breathing. It's not so much of a lung thing, but the sinuses can get stopped up to the point the patient has to breathe through his/her mouth. It can be very difficult. They are thinking about breathing issues and you are wanting them to "poo," so you can get them comfortable again.

At this point, you may have success in rolling the patient to the right side for BMs (and for back care). This right-sided rolling does not challenge the breathing process as much.

The Art of Pooing

Of all the issues associated with caregiving, bowel regulation and bowel movements were my nemesis. If I ever wanted to run far away, it was when we had bowel issues. Why? Two reasons. "Poo Drama" and regularity.

Poo Drama happened when my husband had a total disconnect as to the reality of his situation and insisted that he was going to get out of bed to sit on the commode in the bathroom. I became the bad guy who had to explain that his legs did not work, or I would demonstrate how I had to lift his legs instead of him moving them. I was the one full of bad news.

We tried to uncover his legs so he could see that he couldn't work them (or prove us wrong). Some days nothing worked. He would hold his poo until he could go to the bathroom himself because he was tired of turning to his side to poo. I would have been tired of that, too, but that didn't change the reality of our situation.

There was no magic wand for this dilemma. I looked everywhere!

After a while, the nurse and I agreed that it was time to introduce a medication to address agitation. Haldol helped a bit. Sometimes, I would say that "today" it looked like his legs weren't working, but I *could* roll him to his side. Sometimes I just cheerfully rolled him, ignoring the Poo Drama talk, but nothing consistently worked— especially if constipation was an issue.

I did find something that seemed to help for a while with regularity. A caregiver suggested we try probiotics. I already took them. Maybe my husband, who wasn't eating enough of anything or drinking enough fluids to provide adequate hydration, would benefit? His gut bacteria were surely out of whack.

Well, the daily probiotic helped. Fairly regular BMs resulted that were softly-formed and easy to pass. That sure beat two nights of Milk of Magnesia, followed by many doses of Imodium to stop the diarrhea!

Make sure to discuss all options for bowel regularity with your home health or Hospice nurse. What works for one patient with adequate food, fiber, and fluids will not work for someone barely eating or drinking. The plan you establish for one week, may not work the next, because of the physical decline in your loved one/patient.

Bed Pans Revisited

Born of Poo Drama, the idea of trying the bed pan once again entered my desperate mind. Determined to leave no stone unturned, I tried using the dreaded devise. If there was anything I could do to enhance my husband's pooing experience, I was going to do it! Anything to avoid Poo Drama!

He appreciated the gesture. We gave it a shot. After all, sitting up on a commode-seat-shaped object just might do the trick—in theory.

For us, it was a lose-lose situation. Not only were pooing feelings not enhanced, but his whole backside ended up looking like it had been to a brawl due to the localized bruising from the pressure of sitting on the bed pan.

He was glad to roll on his side to poo again that day though!

Coconut Oil Suppositories and other Helpful Hints

Into the life of every bedridden patient comes concerns about having regular bowel movements.

Aside from the doctor ordering daily stool softeners, Miralax, or Senna-type pills, the occasional impaction may occur. The desire to "go" is there, but nothing will move. You may do a gloved "finger check" of the rectum only to find firm/hard BM.

What to do? Enemas won't work because the fluid will just come back out unchanged.

In such moments, I found a useful home remedy that compliments the use of Senna.

I made coconut oil suppositories. Lacking a mold, I simply took a small piece of aluminum foil and created small, finger-sized troughs. Into these indentations I placed room-temperature coconut oil and put them in the freezer to harden. Once firm, the suppository can be removed from the foil, rolled in your gloved hands to remove any sharp edges, and gently inserted into the rectum of the side-lying patient. One or two can be used if the patient is comfortable with the insertion. Have your nurse show you how to do this safely.

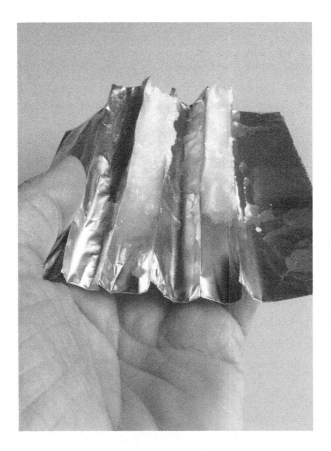

It will take a few hours or overnight, but the BM should emerge, probably totally broken down. I dispensed with the mini-blue pad for such occasions and used half or whole blue pads on top of the one already in place. This will be a multi-step BM process, but the job will be done.

Prevention of constipation is the best cure. You will just have to experiment with what works. In addition to over-the-counter and prescription ordered stool softeners and stimulant laxatives, consider regular consumption of prunes or prune juice.

There is even an exercise for those confined to beds to help stimulate bowel movements.

Using a short length of pool noodle (12 inches long), assist your patient in holding both ends of the noodle, hands placed like end caps, with arms stretched out straight as much as possible. Assist/instruct them to twist his/her arms until they are totally crossed to one side. Hold that position for a few moments. Then they "unscrew" their arms and twist them again in the opposite direction and hold.

This simple side-twisting movement helps to squeeze the core of the body, mimicking normal bowel activity. Repeating this exercise several times, a few times a day, can go a long way in assisting bowel regularity. Check first with your home health or Hospice nurse to see if this would be a safe exercise for your loved one/patient to do.

Helping Bedside Commode Odor Issues

Urine is not our favorite smell, for sure, but BM in a bedside commode can really create a stink bomb. Why? A bathroom toilet can conceal much of the smell of a bowel movement because the deposit is surrounded by water.

It is possible to mitigate some of the smell factor of a bedside commode by keeping some clean water along with a splash of Lysol in the bottom of the removable pan. This is only possible if you can lift the added weight of the water and not slush the contents out when emptying.

Of course, always empty and wipe down the pan with Clorox wipes immediately after using.

Dressing the Bedridden Patient

Without modified clothing, dressing a bedridden patient using anything other than a hospital gown can be difficult for the patient and the caregiver.

The factors of limited range of motion for the patient makes getting shirt sleeves on or off so awkward and even painful.

Then there is the problem of getting the shirt down the patient's back. Often times, the shirt or blouse gets wadded up, pulling on the underarms, or becoming massively wrinkled, causing discomfort and skin breakdown.

To make matters more difficult, the patient probably can't lean forward to help in the dressing process.

What to do?

Some people do an initial modification by slitting the back of the shirt up the center to about 4-6 inches from the neckline. This is the first step in getting arms in sleeves and then popping the rest of the shirt over the head. But there's still the problem of excess fabric and wrinkles starting where the cut ended.

Take things one step further by removing a U-shaped cutout from the back of the shirt, reserving a yolk area to cover the shoulders.

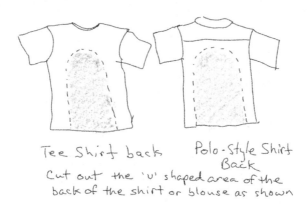

Tee Shirt back   Polo-Style Shirt
Back
Cut out the 'u' shaped area of the
back of the shirt or blouse as shown

This U-shaped cutout leaves enough fabric for total coverage to the sides of the patient's chest and shoulders but does not create wrinkles for him/her to lie on because their back is lying directly on the smooth draw sheet.

My husband looked so dressed up in his modified Polo shirts! He had previously worn long-sleeved button-up shirts but did not need that degree of warmth when confined to bed. Rather than buy a whole new wardrobe from the department store, I went to the nearest thrift store and had a ball selecting Polo-style shirts from racks of great quality options all organized by color. I chose shirts that were a soft knit rather than the rougher waffle knit that some Polo shirts have.

While my experience was in modifying shirts for a man, the concept can be readily adapted for women's shirts, blouses, and night gowns.

DEIDRE EDWARDS

For people who are truly bedridden, additional clothing from the waist down is not needed—they are under a sheet and blanket at all times.

However, if modesty demands—it did for my husband—boxer shorts for a man or a slip or a skirt for a woman can easily be cut for draping across the lap area. We reminded my husband that his "loin cloth" was in place and he was greatly comforted by the added sense of privacy.

So, there *is* more dignified clothing available for your loved one/patient other than the patient gown.

Bathing the Patient

You may need do this for your loved one/patient even if you have the assistance of regular aide visits. Situations arise when you may be called on to do this procedure—or part of it—between visits by aides.

Here are the steps:

———

Bathing the patient by yourself

- Gather the supplies: 4 washcloths, basin, soap (we relied on foaming anti-bacterial hand soap), deodorant, body cream, barrier cream a.k.a. Butt Paste, bath towel, new blue-pad and mini-blue pad if using, and pre-moistened wipes. Put on gloves.
- Fill basin half-full with fairly warm water. Remember, only the wet washcloth is touching the patient, and basin water cools off quickly.

64

- Take basin and other supplies to the bedside table.
- Make sure the bed is at a good working height for you.
- Fold the sheet and blanket down to the patient's waist, remove their shirt (oxygen will have to be temporarily removed to take shirts on/off), and cover their chest with the towel.
- Using only a wet washcloth, wash the patient's face. If they can do this themselves, then give them the opportunity to participate. Otherwise, start with the eyes, wiping from the inner edge of the eye lids to the outer edge. Eyes can get very gunky, so extra attention may have to be paid to this important area. You may have to get a water-only, moistened Q-Tip to gently stroke along the eye lids, twirling the Q-Tip as you move. Please use a fresh Q-Tip for the other eye to prevent cross contamination. Using the washcloth, move on to the forehead, cheeks, nose, and ears.
- Rinse wet cloth in the basin and squirt on some soap. Starting with the arm farthest from you, lift the patient's arm and wash the length of the arm and arm pit with firm but gentle strokes.
- Rinse washcloth out in basin and rinse the arm. Dry it off with a dry washcloth.
- Wet the washcloth and repeat the procedure for the arm nearest you.
- Wet the washcloth, apply soap, then wash and rinse the neck and chest in the same fashion. Make sure the woman's breasts are moved to clean skin under the breast.
- Apply body cream to arms, neck, and chest; and deodorant to the underarm areas.
- Change water if it is too cool or soapy.
- Remove towel from patient's chest and bring covers back up. Pull lower covers up enough to reveal the legs. Place

bath towel under the legs, always lifting extremities with an under-handed "scooping" method and not an over-hand "pinching" grab.

- Wash legs and feet using the same technique as for the arms. Apply body cream. Remove towel and replace covers.
- Change water if it is too cool or soapy.
- NOTE: you are always on the look-out for anything new or unusual about the skin. This is vital as skin conditions can change overnight and without any warning. Skin can go from "great" to "where did *that* come from?" in a blink of an eye. Look under the heels and between the toes for any surprises. Anything unusual will require treating in some way. Consult with your nurse.
- Roll the patient to his/her side using the techniques previously described. Place the bath towel along the length of the bed next to the patient's back.
- Wash the back using long and circular strokes. This is *dessert* for the patient, in a manner of speaking. It feels so good! Also wash the hip area. Dry and apply body cream.
- Using the wipes, wash the anal area and buttocks, discarding the wipes in the trash. Dry and apply appropriate barrier cream. Remove the mini-blue pad, if using, and replace. If the larger blue pad is in good condition, you will not have to change it. If you do have to replace the large pad, using the techniques described in changing an occupied bed, roll the old pad up to the patient's body and tuck under hips. Position the new pad, roll the excess up, and tuck the excess under the rolled-up old pad. Change gloves.
- Return the patient to his/her back and roll to the other side. There's not much left to wash except the side of the back and hip you were not able to reach before. If

changing the blue pads, pull out the old one to discard in the trash and roll out the new one.

- Return the patient to his/her back. Change washcloth and drying cloth. Uncover the genital area and wash, paying close attention to all areas that are skin-on-skin. Women are always wiped "front to back" with a clean section of washcloth for each wipe, with the softer wipes being a better choice for a woman. For men, make sure to get all around the scrotum and between the legs. For an uncircumcised man, the foreskin must be retracted to expose the head of the penis so it can be cleaned; return the foreskin to cover the head of the penis after rinsing.

- All skin folds must be thoroughly dried after washing and rinsing. This means under breasts, between folds of fat on the body, and around the scrotum.

- Bathing is now done. Put a new shirt/blouse on the patient, readjust covers and raise the head of the bed to the desired angle.

- Clean everything up: Put dirty linens in the washer or hang to dry until the next load. Dump the basin water in the toilet. Rinse out with clean water. Wipe the basin with a Clorox wipe. Wipe the over-bed table with a Clorox wipe and the sink area as well.

- Take off gloves and wash your hands. That's it. You're done and deserve to take a break.

———

Drying Skin Folds

As previously mentioned, drying areas where there is skin-on-skin contact is vital to prevent skin breakdown. Sometimes, getting those areas completely dry can be problematic.

Nurses have used hair dryers for years to assist in the drying task, but I wanted something simpler to use that did not require plugging and unplugging.

Behold the hand-held, battery-operated fan. It was perfect for drying skin folds—especially in areas that sweat. I purchased this at Walmart in the summer time; off season, I'm sure there are choices on Amazon.

Keeping Skin Folds Dry

Once those folds are dry ... how do you keep them dry?

You may find that a strip of soft tee-shirt material draped between the folds to be beneficial. These strips can be used in conjunction with any medicated powder that may be prescribed or with simple corn starch.

To make a corn starch shaker out of a Mason jar, punch holes in some waxed paper placed on top and secured with the screw down jar ring.

NOTE: NEVER put Gold Bond Medicated Powder around or near the genital area. It will set your patient on fire! Good on feet maybe, but BAD around private parts. Just saying.

Shampooing hair

Shampooing my husband's hair was a cinch. While the head of the bed is about half-way up, I removed the pillow and placed a bath towel under his head to protect the upper bed and another across the top of his chest.

Working from a pan of warm water, I used a wet washcloth to rub over his head to get his "fringe" and scalp wet. Using a very small amount of shampoo, I washed his head and hair, wetting my hands as needed.

Then, returning to the wet washcloth, I rubbed off the soap. This will require several rounds of rinsing and possibly a change of water.

Dry and style the hair. Remove towels and replace pillow.

Women usually require a different technique because they have more hair. I personally have no experience using those shower caps with dry shampoo, but I hear they are quite effective.

Otherwise, you will need a shampoo tray that sits under the woman's head and drains off into a bucket on the floor. This way, water can be poured over her head before the shampoo is applied. Rinse water is also poured over her head, still draining into the bucket. A towel should be placed under the shampoo tray and another around the woman's neck. Your nurse or aide can walk you through this process and help you acquire a shampoo tray.

Shaving the face

Shaving was fun for me. You see instant results. Whiskers with shaving cream one moment and smooth face the next. What? I didn't use an electric razor on my husband? He had converted to electric years ago and I followed suit for a while, but the results were less than stellar.

Patients on blood thinners are encouraged to use electric razors because of potential bleeding problems if nicks should occur. As long as there are blood thinners on board, you will have to stick with the old Norelco.

But if you are able to use them, nowadays, there are these five-bladed wonders that make shaving with a razor so easy! I love using them on my legs, so I started using the same type of razor to shave my husband's face.

If you do decide to take the plunge to regular shaving with a razor and shaving cream, here are the steps I followed:

———

Shaving a man's face with a standard razor

- Gather your supplies: five-bladed razor, shaving cream, bath towel, washcloth, and bath pan with as warm a water as the patient can tolerate. Remember, we are working with a gently squeezed out washcloth, not direct water contact. You may also get aftershave or a face cream of choice. The wearing of gloves is advised.
- Place the patient in a sitting or near sitting position in bed. Drape the bath towel across the patient's chest, tucking the edges around the neckline, and leaving the extra length of toweling on your side of the bed, which is your drip zone.
- If the patient is wearing oxygen, the oxygen may remain in place for the beard-softening process and then might be removed for the few minutes it takes to shave, if tolerated. Otherwise, you can shave the face with the oxygen in place—you just have to work around the tubing.
- The most important step in a successful shave is in proper softening of the beard. You can't rush or neglect this part. Fold the washcloth in half and dip into the very warm water. Gently squeeze out the cloth so it's not dripping, but is not completely squeezed dry. Place cloth across the beard area, crossing the face just under the nose and still covering the upper lip. This is a caress-the-face time to

keep the cloth in contact with all areas of the beard. When the cloth begins to lose its heat, return it to the basin to rewarm. Repeat this process of beard softening at least three times.

- While the final cycle of beard softening is doing its magic, remove your hands from their caress position and squirt shaving cream onto your non-dominant hand. I am right-handed and was working from my husband's right side. You would need to reverse this if you are left-handed.

- As soon as you remove the warming cloth from the patient's face with your clean, dominant hand and drape it over the side of the basin, apply the shaving cream over the entire bearded area with your other hand. This takes seconds. Then with one clean finger, put a smear of shaving cream just under the nose. Wipe off your finger. Save the lathered hand for future reference as there should be excess lather on your non-dominant hand.

- Dip the razor into the basin, let it drip for a bit, and then start shaving. Start on the far side of the face, just under the side burns, applying gentle but firm pressure. Too light of a stroke will actually not spare the patient from harm; rather, a *whimpish* pressure will tear up their skin. Shave in a downward direction first. You can take several strokes in that area before rinsing the blades off in the water. If the patient's face is *craggy*, you will not be able to shave over the ripples. Use your non-dominant hand to push/pull/manipulate the skin to create a smooth shaving surface.

- Then, using your non-dominant/shaving-creamed hand, run your fingers up and down the shaved area. You can feel any remaining beard. Try shaving in an upward motion. Feel again; you may need to dampen your fingertips as the cream may be drying out. Sometimes a short, sideways stroke may be needed.

- After you have completed the far side of the face and neck, move to the near side.

- The chin area is next. If possible, have the patient roll his lower lip over his bottom teeth to make that area just under the lower lip more accessible. Shave the chin area in a downward motion with shorter strokes. The swivel head of these five-bladed razers makes going over the jaw region and down the neck much more user-friendly. Check your work with the messy hand, chins often need a sideways stroke.

- Lastly, is the mustache area. Again, if the patient can help, ask him to bring his upper lip over the top teeth to smooth out the area. Shave downward, starting right under the nose. Check your work, applying additional cream, if needed, with the messy hand. You will probably need to shave sideways, going toward the center from the side of the upper lip near the mouth.

- Check your work over the whole face with the messy hand. Sometimes creative shaving directions are needed to finish the job, especially at the base of the cheek.

- Finish by rinsing out the washcloth in fresh warm water from the bathroom (the basin water is too dirty with shaving cream and whiskers). Carefully wipe the patient's face clean of any cream residue. Do not forget the mouth, which may have cream trying to get in.

- Apply aftershave or face cream at this time. If you do not want to have your hands smelling like Old Spice for the rest of the day, make sure you are wearing gloves. Trust me on this!

- As you put away your supplies, the basin should not only be rinsed out but also wiped out with a Clorox wipe.

Shaving basins get quite polluted with whiskers and cream.

———

Now, your loved one/patient is feeling all spruced-up and ready to start the day.

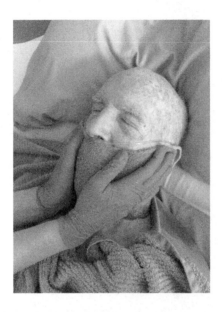

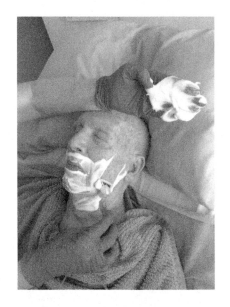

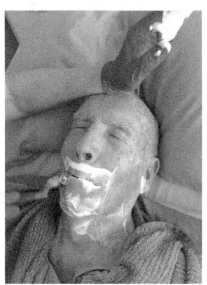

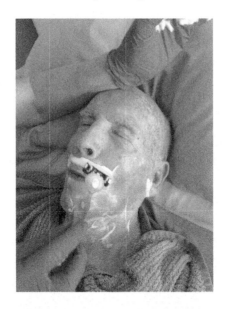

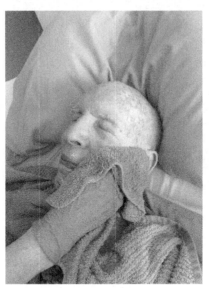

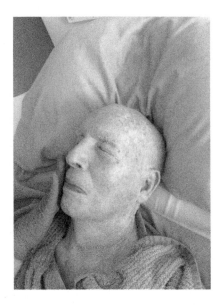

Nail Care for Hands

There's something about not having a lot to do. Idle hands tend to scratch. Fingernails that scratch fill up with dead skin. After just a few days, you'd swear your loved one/patient had gone to the garden to do some serious weeding and had forgotten to wash.

At least once a week—a hand soak, nail clean out, and nail trim are needed. If your loved one/patient is diabetic, always check with your agency's nurse about special precautions.

Here are the steps:

———

Providing nail care

- You will need a bath basin, hand soaps, fingernail clippers, a wooden nail care stick, emery board, paper towel, and hand cream. Nail care sticks are slant-edged wooden implements used to gently clean out the undersides of nails and are available at beauty supply stores, and nail care sections of some drug stores.

- Using a bathing basin, fill with an inch or two of comfortably warm water and a few squirts of anti-bacterial foaming hand soap, and maybe one squirt of a pleasant Bath and Body Works-type hand soap.
- Place a bath towel across the lap of your patient who is sitting up a bit in bed.
- Situate the bath pan so one hand may safely drape into the water without spilling. Have them test the water temperature first with one finger before dunking in their whole hand.
- Gently rub their hand with the soapy water. This can be so relaxing for the patient and provides some quality one-on-one time for you both.
- Because I do not like trimming dirty nails and gumming up the clippers, I prefer to clean under the nails first. To clean the nails, I used the pointy end of the file that swings out from the clippers OR the slant end of the wooden nail care stick. Gently glide the cleaning tool under the nail. Then, after ***each*** swipe, wipe off the tool on the paper towel. A good technique is to do one swipe of each nail, returning each finger to the soaking water as you go. Then, make another pass of all the nails. Repeat until the nails are clean. It can be amazing how much gunk can be removed.
- Now the fingernails are ready to be trimmed with the nail clippers. Care must be taken not to cut the patient. The nails have been soaking and should be softened enough to make things easy.
- Use the emery board to smooth the edges as needed.
- Dry the hand off and place on the towel.

- Repeat for the other hand.
- Apply some cream to both hands when grooming is finished.

———

There you are—happy, clean hands greatly comforted by your loving touch.

Nail Care for Feet

Foot care is not for the faint of heart.

Many people hate taking care of someone else's feet.

If the patient is diabetic, utmost precautions should be taken to not unwittingly create a small cut or nick that could blossom into major problems that, in a worst-case scenario, could lead to an amputation.

Check with your agency's nurse about how to best approach this important point of care. If your loved one/patient cannot leave the house for a visit with a podiatrist, foot care must happen at home.

Don't ignore your patient's toe nails. They won't go away. They will just keep on growing.

I was able to wrap my husband's toes with several rounds of warm washcloths before cleaning, trimming and/or filing his toe nails. I found that cuticle remover/softener liquid does wonders to soften anything above, around, over, or under the toenails before cleaning. A wooden nail care stick is an essential tool for gently scraping off the nail's surface and cuticle, in addition to underneath the nails. Fingernail clippers, generally, will not work for toe nails. Larger toenail clippers may be used.

Again, talk with the nurse about using the proper implements.

Changing the Sheets of an Occupied Bed

Even if your home health representatives or Hospice aides do this for you, chances are very good you may have to do this yourself. While it sounds quite daunting, and maybe contains a trade secret reserved for magicians, you, too, can master this task!

You have already learned how to roll your patient to his/her side. Well, you are practically half-way there!

Here's the whole thing:

Changing sheets while the patient is still in the bed

- Gather your supplies: Clean bottom/top sheets and pillow case, draw sheet, new blue pad and mini-blue pad, if using.
- Remove the blanket but keep the top sheet in place.
- Roll your loved one/patient to his side, preferably to the side the urinary drainage bag is hanging (if using).
- Roll up the exposed blue pads and tuck under the buttocks.
- Next, roll up the exposed draw sheet and tuck under the buttocks and back.
- Undo the fitted sheet all along the free side of the bed, top, and bottom.
- Roll the fitted sheet up to the patient's body, and tuck under their body from head to toe.
- Place the clean fitted sheet onto the exposed mattress,

tucking the remaining clean sheet UNDER everything else that's tucked beneath the patient.

- Next, place the clean draw sheet, rolling/folding up the half that will eventually be on the other side of the bed, and tuck under the patient.
- Then place the clean, full blue pad and roll/fold up the half that will eventually be on the other side of the bed, and tuck under the patient.
- Prepare the patient for rolling back onto his/her back. Tell them there will be a "big bump" or "watch out for the speed bump."
- Roll the patient to his/her back.
- Prepare the patient to roll to their other side. If there is a urinary drainage bag, make sure to temporarily reposition it to the other side of the bed.
- Roll the patient to his/her other side.
- The rest of the old sheets can easily be extracted and rolled up at this point. Separate the blue pads and put them in the trash bag.
- Pull out the clean fitted sheet and finish placing on mattress.
- Then pull out the draw sheet and smooth.
- Finish by pulling out the blue pad and smoothing down all layers for comfort. Add the mini-blue pad at this time, if using.
- Reposition the patient onto his/her back.
- Change the pillow case and place pillow under the patient's head.
- Return the urinary drainage bag to the preferred side.
- The patient is still covered with the old sheet. Place the clean sheet fully on top of the patient, having them hold the top of it. Reach under the fresh one and pull the old one down and out.

———

It's magic! The patient has never been exposed. You can pat yourself on the back. You did it!

Now, I've broken down this task into each small step, so please do not be daunted by seeing 22 of them! It's actually kind of fun.

In practice, the blue pads are changed the most, followed by draw sheets and top sheets. Complete bed changes are just not daily occurrences—depending, of course, on patient needs and conditions. In any case, you now possess "The Secret" and no longer have to feel overwhelmed.

Eating, Drinking, and Feeding Issues

Someone confined to bed is not going to expend the same calories as someone who is ambulatory. Don't be surprised to eventually see a decrease in appetite. Additionally, disease processes can change what is consumed over time.

Sometimes caregivers try to supplement their loved one/patient's dwindling appetite by offering canned or bottled drinks such as Ensure or Boost. They can be a blessing in that they provide both liquid and nutrition. However, the downside can be diarrhea, especially in the formulations that offer boosted nutritional values. You can try their original, basic formulations if the enhanced one is causing problems.

If a nutritional supplement drink results in diarrhea, you can try a protein powder to make a smoothie in the blender. This kind of drink should be user friendly. The good thing is that the flavoring components can be changed up through various fruit ingredients.

For someone with a decreased appetite, reduced portions on

smaller plates seem less intimidating, and you may get a better consumption on their part. There is something about looking at too much food that takes away the little remaining appetite they have.

Make life easier for yourself by **cooking in quantity**. Here are just a few tips I successfully employed:

If bacon is still on the menu, cook the entire package one morning, and stow the extra slices in a zip lock bag either in the fridge or the freezer. I appreciated having to clean up bacon grease spatters only once instead of daily. Reheating cooked slices to sizzling freshness is easy: lay them on some foil in the toaster oven and toast. A medium setting for the toasting process is perfect for refrigerated slices.

Oatmeal. Somehow oatmeal is just so palatable and easy to get down. Good source of fiber, helpful to lowering cholesterol numbers, and an excellent vehicle to ramp up nutritional content. Without fail, I added two large serving spoonfuls of organic coconut oil to this double batch.

Coconut oil is full of goodness and its daily use has been linked to improved cognitive function among other things. I often added ¼ cup or so of Great Lakes Brand collagen hydrolysate, which is a flavorless and bountiful source of protein (11g per 2 rounded Tbs.).

Cinnamon is so yummy in oatmeal and provides great anti-inflammatory properties. Yes, I do use a modest amount of brown sugar when cooking the vat of oatmeal. It doesn't take a huge quantity to gently sweeten a serving.

I cooked a double recipe each time and refrigerated the leftovers in a Pyrex dish with a snap lid. To reheat, I scooped out a desired quantity into a microwaveable dish/bowl. To add creaminess, I sprayed some canned whipped cream on the top of the oatmeal. I set the microwave for thirty seconds or so to reheat. All you have to do is add a handful of blueberries or diced, fresh peaches just before serving. Voila! A power-packed, easy to eat breakfast.

If chewing fried eggs is problematic, but the texture of grits is tolerated, try my *Fluffy Grits*, by cooking a single serving of instant grits and adding one beaten egg, stirring well to incorporate. Microwave the grits a few additional seconds, stir well, and repeat until egg is cooked. With a pat of butter and seasoning, this is a fun treat and can add variety to an easy-to-consume breakfast. A little grated cheese could be added, if tolerated.

Time is tight for most caregivers. This is why cooking in some quantity always plays out well. Leftovers can be arranged to be eaten in the next few days or frozen for future reference.

Not one for packaged foods, I learned to soften my standards by keeping single-serving containers of Jello and different flavored puddings on hand. Formerly, I would have made all of that myself, but time was tight. Additionally, if my loved one/patient's taste buds or culinary desires on a particular day were off, I didn't want an entire recipe of pudding to go to waste until he came around to liking it again. Easier to toss a single serving cup out than a whole recipe I had put effort into making.

Serving meals

The Over-The-Bed Table

One would think placing the over-the-bed table at a right angle to the bed is best; that's how it's usually done.

But you should study the body mechanics of your patient feeding him/herself. If there is awkwardness, rather than ease of natural movements with the over-the-bed table at a right angle, you might find that a different approach creates more accessibility to the plate and cup. Sometimes with a corner of the table aimed at my husband, he showed improved reach and control.

Plates, Cups, and Bowls

A simple solution to securing plates and bowls to prevent them from moving away from the patient is using a piece of shelf-liner grippy stuff under their plates. No longer do they need one hand to eat and another to keep the plate from sliding around the smooth surface of the table.

Pre-cutting meats, French toast, and other foods into bite-sized pieces eliminates the patient needing to use a knife. Cut these items in the kitchen so they can eat what's placed in front of them without having to be helped.

Hospice facilities we have used put all fluids in sippy-type cups with curvy built-in straws. The cup was wavy-sided, which facilitated a secure grip. These cups have a sealed top and would be ideal for shaky hands. I almost ordered some online for home use but didn't. I'm a little nervous about built-in straw sanitation. However, there are probably pipe cleaner-like devices that could address cleaning straws.

What we did for coffee was replace the hard-to-hold and heavier standard ceramic mug with Styrofoam cups. At one point, I discovered my husband would actually drink more fluids if he was using a local BoJangles fast-food coffee cup, which is probably 12 ounces. I'd reuse a cup for several days and then go to BoJangles for another cup of "Joe."

As his fluid consumption decreased, we converted to standard small Styrofoam coffee cups and then to disposable cups with a brown corrugated outer surface. There was less to throw away when he didn't drink it; the cup was lighter to lift, and he didn't have to tip the cup up as far to get the last sip.

For cold drinks such as iced tea, I purchased a plastic, insulated screw-top cup. It also had a solid removable, hard-plastic straight straw. After throwing out the straw, I used colorful flexible disposable straws.

That, too, was replaced with cold drinks being offered in the small Styrofoam or brown corrugated cups, which all had a smaller diameter for gripping and were lighter.

There is a host of adaptive eating equipment for those without full range of motion or grip. Talk to your home health representative or Hospice agency for details about adaptive silverware, plate guards, and cups.

Feeding Someone Else

There may come a time when your loved one/patient is too weak or impaired to feed him/herself. This could be for just one meal or it could become a new reality. Sometimes, you may need to help only with the solid foods if they can still handle the fluids.

Before offering your patient anything to eat—on ANY given day—FIRST assess their ability to swallow liquids. This is easily done with their initial sip of water or beverage before each meal.

Some patients get to the point where drinking liquids becomes difficult, but if those liquids are thickened just a bit, they can be successfully swallowed without choking. You may be able to offer them a tiny bite of pudding or mashed potatoes when they struggle with regular fluids. If this becomes an issue, there are flavorless, powdered thickeners that can be stirred into any liquid. Talk with your nurse about using these.

If choking or serious difficulty in swallowing occurs, contact your nurse before offering any more fluids or foods.

Remember: Difficulty in swallowing fluids means no solid foods and no more fluids. This change in condition must be reported ASAP.

It is generally advisable to punctuate feeding solid foods with offers of some fluids to assist in the general flow of swallowing and digestion.

Meal time is a social time. Sit at eye level as you feed them. Because my husband's hospital bed stayed in the high position, we kept a kitchen stool next to his bed for this purpose, and also for visiting. You may or may not want to eat at the same time yourself, but you can certainly sip on a drink to share in the meal moment.

Smaller bites should be offered. Shoveling food in their mouths to hurry up the process is very dangerous and abusive. Monitor the feeding techniques of any assistant caregivers to protect your loved one/patient from harm.

Brushing Teeth

While denture care is pretty straight-forward according to the products you use, the process of brushing teeth is often over-looked. Granted, around here, brushing teeth was decreased to once a day, right before my husband tucked in for the night, but it is not that difficult of a process if you know what you are doing.

Here are the steps we used:

———

Brushing the patient's teeth

- You will need two plastic cups, a soft toothbrush, tooth paste, and a Kleenex tissue. We used disposable party tumblers that were reused until they need replacing. I put a rubber band around one of the cups to keep it designated as the spit cup. Fill the other cup with cold water.

- Carry the supplies to the bedside table and place the patient in a sitting position.

- Apply the desired amount of toothpaste onto the brush. Dip the prepared toothbrush into the water cup and brush the patient's teeth by brushing the front teeth first to work up a little lather. Then ask your loved one/patient to open his/her mouth. Brush all surfaces of the bottom teeth and top teeth, concluding with another brushing of the front teeth.

- Offer or give a sip of the cold water to swish, which you may need to remind them to do.

- Hold the Kleenex tissue under the spit cup and hold the spit cup directly under their bottom lip so they can spit. You may need to give instructions or encourage them to do this.

- As you withdraw the spit cup, bring the tissue up to wipe their lips.

- You may want to offer a sip of the cold water afterwards.

- Rinse out the toothbrush and the spit cup; throw the tissue away.

Lessons from Chapter 3

There you have it—a complete guide to the basic caregiving skills that are done on a regular basis. That's why these are known as Activities of Daily Living (ADLs).

Your loved one/patient may need special procedures such as urostomy or colostomy care; check with the nurse about how to provide such care and make sure you are thoroughly comfortable in performing those procedures before flying solo.

Remember, a great source of stress for caregivers is feeling inadequately prepared to perform procedures. That's why I am providing you with the free, downloadable, and printable skills shared in this book. Having a step-by-step skill printed out at your elbow should go a long way in ramping up your comfort level. Visit https://deidreedwards.com/index.php/tk4c-bonus-materials/ to access the skills sheets I've prepared for all ***Toolkit for Caregivers*** readers.

Continued guided practice in giving care will result in your loved one/patient's increased comfort, as well as your increased confidence and satisfaction with an ever-increasing skills set. After a while, you will be able to provide care without a second thought.

Coming up next: Some sage advice about priorities and some easy procedures to help organize your efforts and to make your life easier.

4

PROCESSES FOR YOU THE CAREGIVER

While this is not intended to be a "how to cope with being a caregiver" book, I would be remiss if I did not touch on some caregiver-preserving tips. A coping book is needed, for sure, and has just been added to this book! *Love Lives Here: Toolkit for Caregiver Survival* is the bonus book that follows this one. The tips and processes outlined in this chapter will get you started for right now.

Process #1—Regarding Priorities

As the caregiver, your nutritional and psychological status is vitally important. If you collapse, the whole set-up—maybe life itself—could radically change for the worse, for all concerned.

There is a tendency to meet your loved one/patient's needs first, ignoring your own.

Remember what they tell us on airplanes:

"PUT ON YOUR OWN OXYGEN MASK FIRST

BEFORE TRYING TO HELP ANYONE ELSE WITH THEIRS."

It's <u>okay</u> and <u>proper</u> for you to wash **your** face **first** in the morning. If you wash your loved one/patient's face first, you will not take care of yourself at all until noon! Why? Because washing his/her face leads to getting their coffee right away—which leads to getting the newspaper—which leads to heating up that oatmeal—getting their medications...

You see where I am going with this?

Unless you are waking up to a major problem that needs addressing, wash **your** face FIRST.

Process #2—Regarding Sitting Endlessly and Eating Alone

Because my companionship hours with my beloved husband were spent sitting, I found myself sometimes standing up in the kitchen to eat while he slept. It was my body's response to needing to move. The last thing I wanted to do was sit some more while eating by myself.

We usually ate dinner together in his room if he was awake and eating himself, but as his condition changed, I often ate one or two meals without him on a daily basis.

I found it was a welcoming break from eating alone to seek the regular companionship of a friend during meal time whenever possible. Maybe they can bring food, or you can share the cooking experience together. A shared *happy hour* with a beverage, some light snacks, and conversation can really lessen your load.

And remember to never lose any opportunity that provides an extra pair of hands that can help you "oop" your loved one/patient up in bed before the visit ends! I think that every soul who entered our house helped me at one time or another to move my husband up in bed.

I broke up the hours of sitting in his room (reading to him or watching TV at night) with walking tours around the house, getting the mail, or watering the plants briefly outside. My back, legs, and feet all suffered, however, due to this decreased activity —making getting more exercise a daily priority for my preservation.

Prolonged sitting is just not good for you—at the office or while being a caregiving angel—the results are the same.

You must also schedule time AWAY from your caregiving duties, and that time must include body movement, along with a change of scenery.

There is a $10-a-month gym centrally located to my shopping area. Since joining, I managed to go there at least once a week, and often twice. The added exercise and strength training are so rejuvenating and healing. The muscle strengthening is a real plus for caregiving as well.

My chiropractor suggested doing regular lunges throughout the day to stretch those muscles at the hip, which shorten as we sit. Monthly visits to the chiropractor helped, too.

But we can't rely on a doctor to fix us. We have to be creative in eating right, moving our bodies, and stretching muscles. My previous book, ***Toolkit for Wellness- Master Your Health and Stress Response for Life*** has a chapter on home-based exercise ideas that augment its theme of addressing mind-body-spirit wellness. That book is also available on Amazon. ***Toolkit for Wellness*** has helped so many people to a sensible understanding and application of solid nutrition and wellness through its anti-inflammatory approach.

If you are unable to leave the house, simply calling a friend to hear about their life and needs will help you to widen your focus. Such calls are more than venting opportunities for you—they may be crucial as well—and it's so nice to just hear the voice of a friend. Sometimes, you may talk each other off the ledge of life's burdens.

Bottom line—YOU have to be the one to initiate something to help your self-preservation. There are ideas on how to do that in ***Toolkit for Wellness***!

Process #3—Regarding Calendars

Finally! A use for some of those calendars that flood your mail box! Don't throw them away. I'll show you how to put them to good use in organizing your life and in helping remember the patient's status.

Patient Care Calendar

Dedicate one for the patient care area, where you can note any special procedures that have occurred:

- Changing a catheter or urinary drainage bag
- Special medications given: narcotics, laxatives
- Catheter output (if monitoring)
- Abnormal temperatures
- Bowel movements
- Any abnormal occurrence

Now, the little squares on most calendars can't hold that much information. If short-hand notes take up too much space, a supplemental note pad is very handy. Those shopping list pads that also come in the mail with the calendars work perfectly.

You may not need to fill up a calendar or take notes unless your loved one/patient's condition is changing, but a caregiving calendar is a must for remembering the date of the last BM or when a narcotic was given. You think you can remember ... but all that important information runs together after a while. Save yourself some trouble and use a calendar.

These calendars also come in handy during the home visits by the nurse—which will be discussed in the next chapter.

Assistant Caregiver Calendar

The second calendar is for you to note when YOU are going out and WHO is going to take your place.

Unfortunately, spontaneous outings are going to be a thing of the past if you are the sole home caregiver. Everything is scheduled in advance.

Which leads me to a major point: you need to know when to schedule things for **yourself**. Let me recommend that you get coverage for your caregiving duties and schedule a certain day each week that you will be out of the house. That way, there will be no question about when to schedule you next dental appointment, haircut, or lunch out with friends. You already know that, say, Friday is your day out so you can safely schedule meetings and appointments for any Friday.

You will need to get out of the four walls more than that, but one day each week on a set schedule will allow you the liberty of planning in advance and knowing that you are covered.

Getting coverage for yourself can come from several sources:

- An agency
- Individuals you have hired who are qualified
- Helpful friends who will be sitters and not caregivers
- Hospice volunteers who are sitters and not caregivers

There are pluses and minuses to each option.

Some agencies may be unreliable. We used one locally but had to stop because of no-shows. There are good agencies out there but do your homework by talking to people about their experiences with them.

You should also know that agencies charge a hefty hourly fee (around $20 an hour or more for my area) and pay their help a fraction of that fee. It is a business, after all.

I was more successful finding caregivers through the online service Care.com. It's like a dating site, in essence, matching your stated needs with caregiver resumes. You follow-up or not. There is a reasonable monthly fee for this that can be canceled at any time.

Often caregivers know other caregivers, and we were blessed twice because of personal referrals.

By working directly with an individual caregiver, you can set your price above what the worker would get through an agency, but below what an agency would charge you.

There are regulations and laws about tax withholding for hired help. Check with your tax advisor about the details.

If you need to dash to the store unexpectedly, a friend or kindly neighbor can certainly step in for a brief time. However, the concern with this is, what would happen if your loved one/patient needed to have a bowel movement?

This is why I rarely used sitters. If bowels are fairly regulated, having a sitter could be totally fine, and you would not have any concerns. It's just a consideration to keep in mind.

Lessons from Chapter 4

Whether you gradually slipped into the role of being a caregiver or that role was suddenly thrust upon you, the enormity of that new reality usually puts us caregivers into a whirlwind of endless tasks with no sense of direction.

When you apply Process #1 of prioritizing your own care first thing in the morning, you will set yourself up for a properly balanced day and state of mind. Even though your heart puts the needs of your loved one/patient first, you must actually keep yourself going first. Remember—if you are constantly neglecting yourself, you will become so worn down that you will be incapable of being the kind of caregiver you want to be.

Process #2 reminds you of the importance of combatting endless sitting and social isolation and addresses the often-neglected aspects of vital caregiver needs. Becoming more physically active and satisfying your own social needs are as valid of a priority as the needs of your loved one/patient. You must understand that the health and well-being of both of you is a symbiotic relationship. You are intertwined and rely on each other. In a Hospice situation, the health of your loved one/patient is declining but yours must not. You must thrive as best you can in order to be there for them.

In longer sustained declines, keeping your spirits up requires consistent effort on your part in scheduling outings, proper coverage for your absence, and in calling in friends for visits during your meals. Calling friends when you are hanging on by a thread will also go a long way in keeping your spirits buoyed and above water.

Process #3 of using calendars revolutionized my daily organization. As caregiving concerns and observations of decline rent at my heart and created *fuzzy brain*, I simply relied on my calendars and notes. Writing down events and scheduling coverage for my absences were tools that made my life go so much smoother.

I am certain that these tips will help you, too.

Next, we will cover what happens during home visits from the home health or Hospice agency, and how using calendars will help everyone during those visits as well.

5

PROCESSES FOR HOME VISITS

Given the typically blurry nature of an overwhelmed caregiver's mental focus, the parade of people coming in and out of your home may seem random—you can't see the organization or meaning to it all. Keep reading. All will be made clearer right away as I describe the various personnel who may be helping you and your loved one/patient.

Your home health organization or Hospice agency will provide regular home visits from nurses, aides, therapists, social workers, and chaplains.

The **nurse** will check:

- Vital signs
- Skin condition
- Date of last BM (Remember the calendar!)
- Urine amount and quality
- Dressings/bandages
- Comfort and pain levels

- Food intake
- The need for any additional medicines or supplies

This is the time to share your patient care calendar information and any supplemental notes you have taken. This will really help the nurse as she/he discusses with you and the patient the plan of care based on current needs. They can give you helpful hints and answer your questions. The home health and Hospice nurse is also a great resource for information and comfort for you, the caregiver, too.

Nursing visit frequency will depend upon the patient's status. Home health visits may be just monthly; whereas, Hospice visits were twice a week for us. As the patient's condition declines, even daily visits may be needed.

In case of death, the nurse is called in to pronounce the patient's death and will assist the family with closure and in contacting the funeral home.

Nurse aide visits will help you with the patient bathing process. A full bed-bath may not be needed every day, and you may not need help doing that task every time. We had daily help from an aide at the beginning, and then later, we had help twice a week. I handled any in-between bathing needs, along with daily face shaving, regular fingernail and toenail cleaning and trimming, haircuts, and shampoos. This is something you work out with your aide and nurse.

Every situation is different. Some caregivers prefer daily aide help in either getting their loved one/patient started for the day or for the going to bed process. Not all caregivers can do the work needed for a complete bed bath.

All efforts should be made on the home front to expedite the ease of your aide's visit, no matter how frequent. Your home health representative or Hospice aide is probably seeing six, seven, or eight patients a day, and possibly traveling over 100 miles daily to do this.

Answer your phone when the aide calls to confirm an arrival time. If no one responds to their call, how can they be sure someone will be at home to receive them? Common courtesies go a long way to smooth communication and to getting the job done.

Keep bathing supplies together including: soaps, hand sanitizers, Clorox wipes, gloves, plenty of clean washcloths, towels, clean draw sheets, bed linens, and blue pads. Having supplies readily at hand means the aide can spend more relaxed time with your loved one/patient rather than having to search the house for scarce supplies.

Social worker visits are for both the patient and caregiver. Visits by the Social Worker were at least once a month for us. They can help with ideas for community resources that may assist you. They also focus on how the patient and caregiver are coping with life. The Hospice social worker will help coordinate any transfers to a Hospice facility for respite, acute, or residential care.

Respite care is available to caregivers when *they* need a break. It is possible to take up to a five-day break every few months, whereby the patient is transported to an available Hospice facility if there is an opening.

We did that once so I could fly out of state for our daughter's graduation from residency. My husband and I agreed, I was not to miss that event. I had to represent both of us. It was great not having to worry about his welfare for a few days.

Having said that, it might have been better to have kept him home with private duty or agency help 24/7. There would have been less confusion, perhaps, without a change of scenery—but, on the other hand, the main confusion was due to my not being there. You do what you have to do with the resources available to you at that moment. That's where the social worker helps.

Physical or Occupational Therapist visits may be ordered by the doctor if there is still a chance for further improvement in mobility or in participation in self-care. The number of visits depends upon the patient's progress. Such visits may include exercises to strengthen muscles for body movement or to reinforce fine motor skills used in ADLs (Activities of Daily Living). These visits are for home health patients only. Hospice patients, by definition, are not seeking improvements but rather comfort measures.

Pastoral care visits will be offered, which can help both the patient and caregiver with the spiritual adjustments that follow becoming homebound and/or bedridden. Whether or not you are affiliated with a faith-based group or organization, such visits can help because the pastoral care staff is well-versed in home healthcare and Hospice needs.

Lessons from Chapter Five

Visits from the home health or Hospice agency personnel provided a veritable life line to me as a caregiver. Each one of them became a vital cog in my wheel of sanity and, of course, were also a highlight to my husband's day.

Organizing your home medical supplies in a handy, predictable location will be a blessing to these visiting angels. Using a patient calendar and notes for changes in your loved one/patient's condition will free you from straining your memory and will give the nursing providers with a written reference for their notes as well.

Each home visit provides yet another reminder that you and your loved one/patient are not alone on this journey. There is professional help available. What a comfort!

6

BRING THE PARTY HOME

I am not trying to make light of the seriousness of having your loved one/patient confined to bed or being under Hospice Care, but remember what I said in the beginning? The room that your loved one/patient is confined to is their WORLD.

I believe we live until we die. So, as much as possible, bring the party home—to their room.

This chapter will highlight various ways you can bring life to someone whose world has become four walls. Not only will what you do help brighten your loved one/patient's world, but it will also brighten yours. Everyone wins when spirits are lifted.

Hallmark Moments

If you have ever seen a Hallmark movie, you know their movie sets depicting home interiors are always tricked out to the max for any given season. Well, I "Hallmarked" my husband's room up good for the holidays!

When my church choir had its party for Christmas, I volunteered to have it at our house. People were delighted to take turns going in to visit my husband, eat together, and enjoy the decorations. We capped the night off by serenading him with Christmas Carols. He even joined in! What a moment!

There was always a seasonal garland or creative battery-operated string of lights on the bureau, and flags or wreaths hanging on closet doors—you name it.

If your loved one/patient is able to partake in a happy hour-type event with beverages (non-alcoholic or otherwise) and light snacks, bring it on! Gather family and friends around his/her bed and share a laugh.

I cherished the pre-dinner awake times with my husband as we shared a cup of coffee, soda, or tea and I read to him until it was time to get our dinner together.

Make everyday events as special as possible through your presence, cheerfulness, and in your efforts to bring the world to them.

Reading the newspaper can be a joint event. Your loved one/patient may look at the paper on his/her own, but you can read aloud the articles that catch your interest that might have been missed. My husband actually preferred having things read to him—and we never missed the comics!

I know, just the sound of our voice is calming to our loved one/patients. They may be in and out of sleep or consciousness, but they can still hear our voice. When I sometimes stopped to take a sip to rest my voice for a moment from reading aloud, my seemingly asleep husband would open his eyes and ask if I was going to continue.

The sense of hearing is so strong and is the last thing to go, so be careful what you say, even at the bedside of someone in a coma. Reading, singing, and listening to favorite music can all bring a balm to their soul.

I think that total silence around the clock would be so disorienting to someone in an altered state. Sounds give us something to "hang our hat on" ... to ground us to the here and now. Sound helps us tell day from night.

You will be able to tell if your loved one/patient wants a little peace and quiet, and that should be honored.

If they are still conversant and alert, include them in asking advice about or in discussing (non-upsetting) family or world issues. It's such a compliment to them to be asked an opinion and to still seek their wisdom.

We were fortunate enough to bring a TV into my husband's room. We were able to share in watching our favorite shows while we held hands. A radio and CD player can bring the world of music and memories to lift spirits.

Family picture albums can be revisited—if seeing old photos is not upsetting. Those with serious dementia reach a point where looking at pictures of people they do not recognize can be disturbing and create agitation.

Viewing the current Facebook feed usually always includes some viral thread of cute kids or animals to lighten the moment and elicit a laugh.

A favorite pastime of ours was watching the many kinds of birds at our bird feeder on the porch. That ended when my husband became confined to our bedroom. Our son and his family found him a bird feeder that suctioned onto our bedroom window. It was so fun to watch the birds discover this additional feeder. Birds...and yes, squirrels who "rob" bird feeders ... are such an endless source of entertainment.

Various types of garden stakes with hangers for bird feeders are readily available to bring bird watching to any garden area that can be viewed from a window.

All of these activities help the caregivers as well. A cheerful environment is good for everyone.

If you do not have the time, energy, or strength to do some of these things, then speak out. Share your needs with the many people who want to help you but who don't know what to do.

Give them a little task: Could they help cheer up your loved one/patient's room with seasonal decorations? People would fall all over themselves doing that.

Could they read to your loved one/patient while you take a nap?

Could your church put up a bird feeder outside the bedroom window?

That's one thing a caregiver must learn to do. Speak out. Call someone. Maybe just the sound of someone else's voice on the line will be what you need. Don't assume that your friends know when you are having a needy moment or a bad day. Speak out. Save yourself.

Lessons from Chapter 6

You need to survive ... no ... more than that ... you need to *flourish* as best you can under the current circumstances. Making things cheerful as possible in their room, punctuating your caregiving duties with regular outings, bringing the party home, and speaking out when in need, all go a long way to not only helping your loved one/patient but in helping you.

There are a few odds and ends I wanted to make sure to share with you in the next chapter, so let's get started.

7

ODDS AND ENDS

These are some additional tips that need to be shared. A little random, perhaps, but definitely noteworthy.

DNR orders

If your loved one/patient is on Hospice care, there will be a Do Not Resuscitate (DNR) order in place. Hospice care is geared toward keeping a patient as comfortable as possible, free from extreme life-sustaining measures, so that they may die with dignity. A DNR order means that no resuscitation measures will be taken to bring them back from dying.

Many people who are not on Hospice care also have DNR orders.

The thing to remember about having this one-page document, which must be signed by the doctor, is that it must accompany the patient wherever he/she goes. If there are medical appointments or a trip to the Emergency Department, it must go with them. If they transfer, even briefly, to a Hospice facility for respite care, the DNR goes with them.

Always keep the DNR order readily accessible; do not file it away in a drawer. Many people keep them on the refrigerator door or on a table by the front door.

Make sure ALL caregivers and sitters know to NOT call 911 if your loved one/patient dies while they are on watch. Instruct them to call the home health or Hospice agency, and you, in the event of death. The agency's phone number should be readily available—probably on a magnetic sticker on the refrigerator.

Keep Supplies Handy

I cannot emphasize too much how important it is to keep patient care supplies handy. The top of our dresser held folded sheets, mini —and full—blue pads, bath towels, barrier cream, and pre-moistened wipes. The nearest bathroom held the ever-useful bath basin, and all bathing and hygiene supplies were kept inside of that. There was a stack of fresh washcloths folded on the top back of the commode. Paper towels, hand sanitizer, and hand soaps were next to the sink.

There will be other medical supplies as well such as extra briefs, wipes, creams, tubing, and anything else your home health or Hospice agency orders for your loved one/patient. Try to keep these in an easy-to-access location known by all who would need them.

Time seemed to always be tight for the Hospice aides, and nurses. Do everyone a favor by keeping supplies handy.

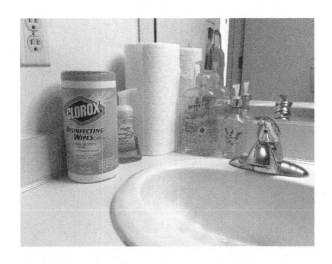

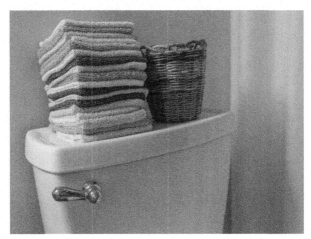

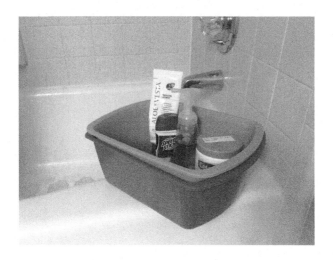

Help for Unhappy Toes

Sometimes toes just don't like touching each other.

We had a phase in which we wove a folded Kleenex around my husband's toes. That worked okay, but another trick really helped when just one toe was irritating its neighbors. I took a super large cotton ball, pulled out the center, and placed the resulting "donut" around the offending toe. Worked perfectly.

Power Outages

If your loved one/patient is using a room air concentrator for supplemental oxygen or if you want to keep the electric bed powered during a storm, it is advised to get on a priority list with your electric company.

Our power provider has a downloadable/printable form the doctor needs to sign and then be turned in to them in order to have our household put on a power priority list. Being on such a list will not guarantee that your house will be the first to regain power during an outage, but it helps for them to know your needs in advance.

The health care agency you are using will contact the oxygen equipment supplier to arrange for extra oxygen canisters to be delivered to your home prior to approaching storms. It's such a comfort knowing there are back up supplies in case of power outages.

Call your electricity provider way before storm season for their particular requirements.

Hurricanes and Other Natural Disasters

An approaching violent storm takes on new meaning when considering the safety of someone significantly impaired or confined to a bed. Home health and Hospice agencies go into overdrive when there is a chance for any kind of disaster. The Social Worker will coordinate with the caregivers well in advance of storms regarding temporary emergency transfers to facilities in safer locations.

Anticipating the location of a safer area is an imperfect science. Knowing exactly where a storm will hit or where the flood waters will flow is nearly impossible; but every effort will be made to transfer your loved one/patient to safety. Doing this requires vast organization and ADVANCED notice.

Changing your mind from hunkering down for the storm to "we need help" at the last minute is not cool. Finding available beds and transportation to another town cannot be done instantly. Generally, Hospice facilities have sleeping chairs or couches for families who want to stay with their loved one/patient; but in a pinch, the patient may have to be relocated to a nursing home until it's safe for him/her to return home.

Separating loads of laundry

It might be a good idea to keep your loved one/patient's laundry separate from everyone else's. It's a Standard Precautions thing. The linens, washcloths, towels, and clothing of your loved one/patient should be washed and dried by themselves. Doing an empty wash load with a bit of bleach between their loads and others might be helpful as well.

Inappropriately Twinkling Eyes

We all like to see that spark of life and a twinkle in the eyes. Good for everyone. But sometimes there comes a twinkle that says other things ... a definite *come hither* look. Okay with a spouse, but not okay with a cute 20-something caregiver, or a 45-year-old Hospice nurse!

Don't blush with shame or mortification at what your loved one/patient is doing. Our sexual sides die only when we die. I've seen sweet little old ladies and men get totally inappropriate with those around them from time-to-time.

Disease processes, physical deterioration, and being confined to bed are all wreaking havoc on hormones and the self-control centers in the brain. The problem is not so much that your loved one/patient is getting fresh or inappropriate, the problem is how the caregivers handle it.

An all-business attitude helps. When your loved one/patient has that extra *sparkle*, just tell them their words and actions are inappropriate. Nobody likes it when they do *that*. If they continue with such words or actions, the caregiver will leave the room except for necessities. Remind them, their spouse/family member does not like it when they do that either. If touching or grabbing is the issue, stay out of their reach.

I have seen such issues come and go. Some days it is an issue, and others it is not even on the radar. Talk with the home health representative or Hospice nurse if this becomes a regular problem. There are medications that may help.

Lessons from Chapter 7

In trying to create as complete of a caregiving picture as I could, these seemingly random items had to be included.

From DNR Orders and Hurricane issues, to *twinkling eyes,* there's so much to consider. I did not want to leave a single thing out in hopes you could feel as prepared as possible.

So many major life events do not come with a hand book: Getting married, how to raise a child, caring for people at home. There are some advice books on a few of these things—marriage and child raising—but not so much on how to actually take care of someone confined to home or confined to bed. Now you have one.

I sincerely hope that I have covered most of the bases for your caregiving journey.

8

IN CONCLUSION

Each situation is unique. I lived through mine, not yours. I just hope that something I have shared in this little book has helped you in the very big life-adjustment of having a loved one/patient confined to a hospital bed at home.

Whether it is over a short or a long period of time, a certain skill set is acquired. Unfortunately, that usually happens by trial and error.

With the resources you have been given in this book, you will, hopefully, not have to fumble in the dark through that unknown maze without a map or a flashlight. After reading and employing some of the tips I've talked about, you should feel well-equipped with skills that will light your way through the world of caregiving.

I was so blessed to have had a loved one/patient who was pleasant, thankful, patient, cooperative, and ever so appreciative of everything I did. That is an exception to the rule, probably. You may be faced with someone who is confused, demanding, and grumpy.

But, in spite of it all, aside from being exhausting—being a caregiver is an honor, a humble privilege, and a personal growth opportunity unlike any other.

Coping with being a caregiver is the stuff for another book—and as a BONUS to you <u>Love Lives Here: Toolkit for Caregiver Survival</u> follows next. Keep reading!

My hope is that now, you have a few skills and tricks under your belt, you will feel more confident in your daily ministrations and will feel less drained and frustrated. If so, my task is done.

THANK YOU READERS

It's probably quite unusual to write most of a book in thirty days while being a caregiver, but that's what I did. In the middle of caring for my beloved darling of 42 years, I was moved by God's inspiration to help others by writing this.

While it has taken me over another year to get it finalized, I consider this a gift. God's gift of inspiration for me to write it, and God's gift of hope and guidance for you—as you to read and use it.

Thank you for choosing to read this book. Thank you for telling others about the helpful information contained here.

If you purchased through Amazon, I would love your feedback through a thoughtful review!

Additionally, I invite you to follow my blogs at foodtalk4you.com and deidreedwards.com where topics are discussed that address health issues, "one bite, one breath, one movement at a time."

Feel free to contact me at deidre@toolkitsforhealth.com for any questions, concerns, or information about: Designed for Health or Caregiver classes; presentations to groups; or discounts for bulk orders of this book for your group, business, or organization.

ACKNOWLEDGMENTS

First of all, to God be the glory! I could never have become as proficient a caregiver as I was without His leadership and guidance every day in my life. He gave me the best man in the world to be my beloved husband, and I thank Him for guiding me every step of the way in being a loving caregiver to him.

My husband, Virgil, was totally supportive in this new undertaking of writing another book. It was in doing and trying everything possible to make myself a more capable caregiver, that he received my daily ministrations. Some things worked, some things didn't; but Virgil remained cheerful and supportive of everything I did to make his life as full and comfortable as it was.

Thank you, darling! Always and forever!

Our dear children, James and Serena, thank you for your patient support and the balance you bring to my life. You were there through thick and thin—patiently listening to too much information, providing emotional and mental support, and frequently being here physically, even though you live hundreds and thousands of miles away. You both could add editor and proofreading skills to your resumes!

Our Hospice team kept me going through thick and thin. They provided a never-ending source of encouragement and support, not only for what was going on with my husband and me, but for this dream I had of helping others through the writing this book.

I want to list just a few of the many people we were blessed with in two years of Hospice care; I know I have left someone out, but thank you to nurses: Donna Rinehart, Brandy Short-Coleman, Ann Marie Golombeski, Sherry Holler, and Marie Wellmer. Thank you to aides: Tamara Cross, Brenna Zamarripa, Heather Gray, Elaine Phillips, and Taquaia Bryant. Our social worker, Shakinna Rodgers, was so helpful in our journey, too. Just know that 3HC (Home, Health, and Hospice Care) has my heart.

I will be forever connected to a very special circle of caregivers who helped me out and allowed me to have a life outside of the house. Nichole Wilson, Brittany Weber, Melissa Opphile, Brenda Mayberry, and Lynne Agnew. You were my lifeline and special friends to Virgil. I wouldn't have trusted Virgil's care to anyone else. You were a part of the love that lived in our house.

The loving soul-support and kindnesses of my church choir, Amen and Overby Sunday School Classes, church members, and pastoral staff of First Baptist Church, New Bern, North Carolina, kept both our spirits buoyed up, and encouraged me throughout the book writing process. Every visit came at just the right moment.

My dear friends and neighbors, Zelda Dardzinski, Carole and Reuben Hart, Greg and Anna Pearson, and Karen Dafonseca kept me sane with visits, phone calls, listening ears, shared glasses of wine, and hugs.

Elaine Varley stepped out of her comfort zone as a professional nature photographer to take pictures of modifications I made to Virgil's bed, as well as other caregiving items. You were so gracious to do that. One of Elaine's amazing sunflower photos brightened Virgil's world and was one of his favorites to look at. Elaine's Nature Photography can be viewed at www.elainevarley. zenfolio.com.

Sheree Alderman—besides being my editor, you talked me off the edge more than once. Our lengthy chats while I paced the yard trying to take in sunshine and fresh air during Virgil's naps, meant so much to me -you'll never know. What a dear friend and encourager at all times.

Special thanks to my beta readers Betty Eliopulos and Hope Dees. My launch team was crucial in getting this book off the ground. You all have my heart and undying gratitude. Thanks.

ABOUT THE AUTHOR

After writing her first book, **Toolkit for Wellness—Master Your Health and Stress Response for Life**, Deidre had no idea that her next book would be about caregiving. She had already learned to embrace new opportunities to help others—regardless of their needs—so a change from personal wellness and stress management to home caregiving techniques was a natural shift.

When her husband's long physical decline resulted in his being placed under Hospice care, Deidre imagined that all that she had experienced through being a nurse and an instructor for Certified Nursing Assistants would certainly come into play. What she hadn't counted on was the big learning curve that would be involved.

As Deidre acquired and invented tricks-of-the-trade to make her husband more comfortable and her role of caregiver easier, the teacher in her began to formulate an idea. After nearly 20 years as a Registered Nurse and National Board-Certified teacher in Career and Technical Education/Health Sciences, Deidre saw an opportunity to lower the anxiety levels for the over 35 million caregivers nationwide, who must surely feel as overwhelmed as she sometimes felt.

Deidre's hope is that, through sharing what she has learned as a home caregiver for a bedridden loved one/patient, her readers will be saved from their feelings of being massively overwhelmed by the unknown. Her conversational style and humor will help the readers feel they are not alone, and they do not have to re-invent the wheel. She provides the guiding light.

Disclaimer: Deidre would like to remind her informed readers that each caregiving situation is unique. She is not claiming to cover all possibilities or circumstances. She encourages her readers to use this **Toolkit for Caregivers,** in conjunction with working with their own home health organization or Hospice professionals.

Deidre continues to write about wellness on her blog, foodtalk4you.com, and holds *Caregiver* and *Designed for Health* wellness seminars as described on her business page at DeidreEdwards.com.

For comments or to book a *Designed for Health* or *Caregiver* seminar, contact Deidre by email at deidre@toolkitsforhealth.com. You are also encouraged to contact Deidre about discounts available for bulk purchases of this book for your business, group, or organization.

IN MEMORIAM

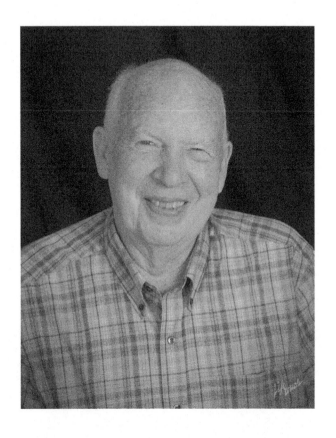

Virgil J. Edwards
1934-2018

Love Lives Here

Toolkit for Caregiver Survival

For before, during, and after

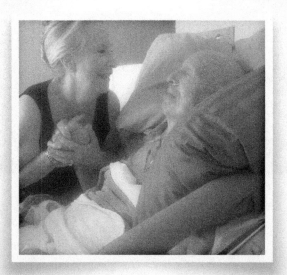

DEIDRE EDWARDS

LOVE LIVES HERE

A TOOLKIT FOR CAREGIVER SURVIVAL …
FOR BEFORE, DURING, AND AFTER

*This book is dedicated to everyone who has ever been,
or whoever will become, a caregiver to a loved one.*

FOREWORD

Learning how to do the actual skills of caregiving for your loved one is covered in the companion book to this, ***Toolkit for Caregivers—Tips, Skills, and Wisdom to Maximize Your Time Together***.

Do you realize that the seeds to ***surviving*** caregiving actually are planted ***before*** your first loving ministrations are given?

This book can, in essence, be the ground work on which caregiving survival can be built upon, many years or decades before the need arises. Hopefully, you'll get to read it that far in advance.

Even if you are already in the middle of taking care of a loved one, rest assured, ***Love Lives Here: Toolkit for Caregiver Survival...For before, during, and after*** will help hold your hand through the roller coaster journey that challenges millions of people every year.

You will experience the following things:

- The normal fears of the unknown will be lessened as a plan for survival is mapped out.
- Learning from the wisdom of others will not only show you that you are not alone, but will also give you hope.
- Knowing what may lie ahead will give you some idea on how you may adapt and prepare.
- A simple check list will assist you starting immediately after your loved one dies.
- Your life-long journey of grief should take on a softer, gentler focus as you apply the re-framing processes learned here to your new circumstances.

As surely as we are born, we are going to die. We will be greatly blessed as caregivers if we can not only do the job if called upon, but also survive—no, flourish—during and after our loving care.

Keeping our caregiver spirits up may be the biggest challenge of all. The help in this book is designed to do just that.

DISCLAIMER

The information shared and expressed in this book is based on the author's own experiences and from interviews with her local representative from the Clerk of Court's office.

The author encourages her readers to seek the advice and guidance from their own legal counsel and Clerk of Court's office regarding all legal matters pertaining to Advanced Directives, Powers of Attorney, estate planning, Last Will and Testaments, and probate matters.

Deidre also encourages her readers to maintain close contact with their medical and mental health professionals who can assist them through the challenges and adjustments with being a caregiver and in coping with grief. Her advice is based upon personal experience, not from a standpoint of being a physician or a licensed mental health practitioner.

The author assumes no responsibility for the results of anyone applying the recommendations she shares here.

INTRODUCTION

It's that shell-shocked, what's-coming-next look. I had it. You may have it right now.

- "When will my loved one's deterioration stop? Is this going to go on and on? One crisis after another?"
- "How am I going to go on if he/she can't function like normal?"
- "How can I last another day?"
- "What's going to happen to us? ...to me?"

Is any of this striking a cord with you? I saw these thoughts and emotions reflected in the face of a friend the other day. I knew that look. It had been mine not long ago. Definitely time for a reassuring hug and an offer to lunch.

As someone who has gone into the storm, weathered it, and come out on the other side, I want to help you do the same. Help you keep your head above the raging waters that threaten to undo all of us caregivers.

You know, it's not an easy process. We are exhausted physically, mentally, and emotionally. Moreover, caregiving is, more often than not, tied up in the deterioration and the death of a dear loved one. Take any stress evaluation test you want, we caregivers are pegging the needle on the stress gauge.

Crawling out of this caregiving storm like a battered and bruised warrior on his/her last breath, should not be the goal. That's bare minimum survival and not a recipe for a long life.

You can aim higher than that and I'll show you how.

We caregivers fall into a particular category of those living with grief. While every grief story is unique, those of us who have lovingly given care to someone dear to us—someone in our home—we have experienced some degree of anticipatory grief that definitely colors how we grieve after we have hung up our caregiving wings.

Grief is not something we shed over time. We learn to live with it.

Our loss starts out consuming the entire canvas of our life. In time, it can still occupy space on that canvas, but it will become smaller by varying degrees—allowing for other aspects of life to be painted in around it.

Let me start this survival guide by exploring the nature of the love that unites you to your loved one, and how nurturing that bond will help your own caregiver experience.

1

LOVE IS

Being someone's caregiver is born of love. Regardless of familial relationships or deep friendships, caring for others springs from the love you share with them. It's the love that drives the whole thing. Period.

But what about love? "How does love have anything to do with my being a caregiver?" you may ask. Consider the following.

Love Is...

- Carefully and lovingly crafted, giving every consideration to another—and yet...
- It is natural, not forced, and flows from the heart, soul, and mind.

The result is a beautiful, sparkling edifice that can be felt and seen. An atmosphere of love creates an almost physical presence that even casual onlookers can notice.

Okay. So now what? Well ...

Somebody's going to go first. We are never assured who that will be; so **love dictates** mutual preparedness.

The same way parents will bundle up their children before letting them outside on a cold, windy winter's day, potential caregiving couples will want to prepare each other for life's eventual storms.

It's that love again.

Whether you are the husband or wife, child or parent, brother or sister, or best friends, love should... no **must**... guide the desire to have the direct personal conversations that will mutually prepare ALL concerned **when...** not if... the need arises.

———

Take-Aways from Chapter 1:

- What are the reasons for you becoming a caregiver? Because you care about someone; you love them.
- Love naturally causes us to look down the road to prepare for the unexpected and to forestall problems affecting our loved one and us.
- Start thinking how helping each other prepare for the future is the natural expression of your mutual love.

2

BEFORE THERE IS A NEED

We do not know when a need will arise.

"But we've got lots of time. We're all healthy. Talking about someone getting sick and dying is depressing! We'll do that later."

If we are really building love and consideration, the get-around-to-it avoidance must be replaced with action.

Doing nothing is not a reflection of love and consideration, but rather a denial of the eventual need that comes to us all. Are you really willing to put the extra burden of being clueless in a crisis on everyone's plate?

A total reversal of life as we know it often happens in a most unexpected instant. Everyone's suffering will only be compounded if all parties are not prepared.

Is your current plan, no plan? Let love and consideration be your guide to taking action.

Next, we'll explore how to prepare for the future.

The Conversation

"The Conversation" is a great way to start. Is this going to be awkward? With love, it shouldn't be. In fact, this conversation should be repeated and expanded to include a wider circle of family (or friends) so everyone will be on the same page.

Try this:

"Honey, when something happens to me, there are some things I want you to know about. I also want to know about some things you do all the time so I'll be prepared if something happens to you first."

The following list should get the conversation rolling:

Advanced directives: Living will

Are you young and healthy? Chances are, you'll want all possible medical interventions done to preserve your life.

Are you 98 years old? Maybe you want to die a natural death with no interventions.

Did you know the medical community is bound to do all that's possible to *bring you back*? That is, unless you have your wishes put on paper, notarized, and others are made aware of your directions.

As long as you are able to hobble or roll into a doctor's office, they will set you up for all kinds of appointments, tests, and therapies. Maybe you are weary of all of that and just want to spend your dwindling strength enjoying sitting in the sunshine.

If that is the case, start a dialogue with your family and doctor about a plan of care designed to support your comfort issues; perhaps a Do Not Resuscitate (DNR) order may be your desire.

What about if you are young and healthy but have been declared brain dead as the result of an accident? Do you want to be kept alive with a ventilator and tube feedings even if you will never wake up?

Most people have firm beliefs about such topics, having discussed them thoroughly around the coffee table at home; but nothing has ever been put down on paper in an official way. This is the stuff of headline news stories depicting the desperate family sagas of differing opinions, splitting loving families apart.

Put your love into action by making your wishes known to all, so that when you no longer have a voice, your desires will still be carried out as you intended.

Are you an organ donor?

Is there a card in your wallet or a designation on your driver's license? If not, no one will know. If something happens to you, save your family making a decision about that by making your wishes known—officially—in advance.

Advanced Directives: Legal and Medical Power of Attorney

If something happens and you are unable to give consent to medical care because of your condition, who is your designee? If you have no family, who do you want to speak on your behalf for medical wishes? Who will manage your estate after you die if you have no family?

Make your wishes known by designating a Medical and a Legal Power of Attorney. Even married couples with children do this. An attorney can help you with these designations

Last Will and Testament

No matter the size of your estate, making plans to distribute your assets just makes sense. Assuming your relatives will fairly decide who gets what, is the stuff of fairy tales—and has set up families for permanent divisions and bad feelings.

Again, show your love for all by clearly expressing your wishes—preferably using an attorney, or at least by having your Last Will and Testament signing witnessed and notarized—and take the guessing out of what will happen to your possessions.

Funeral plans

Another get-around-to-it-someday-soon favorite. There's enough to do when someone dies that—in loving consideration—we should definitely NOT want to add to our survivor's burdens by making them plan and pay for arrangements at the time of our death.

Burial or cremation? That's the first choice. From here, there is a lot to be discussed, planned, and paid for. You'll shower your survivors with countless blessing by having as much as possible planned and paid for in advance.

Bank Accounts with right of survivorship/transfer on death

These are delineations that are generally communicated to the banking institution when accounts are established. If you are uncertain how your account is set up, just ask the next time you are at the bank. If not, accounts may have to clear the probate process before things are settled.

Titles to houses, cars, boats, etc.

Even if there are two names on a title, the property may have to go through a probate process if there is no designation on it that specifically says joint ownership with right of survival. These specifications are easily made at the time of purchase but can be changed through the titling agencies. To avoid a probate process, make sure rights of survivorship are clearly indicated on all titles.

Credit Cards

If a married couple, the caregiver would do well to already have a credit card solely in his/her name, because jointly owned credit card accounts will have to be closed (upon death of a spouse) and the survivor will have to reapply for a new card. It would be nice to not face that process while grieving.

Insurance policies

House, car, health, and life insurance policies' content and location must be known by all concerned. How often are the policies paid? What do they cover?

Past tax papers

Knowing where the old tax documents are located is a great start for survivors in preparing the current year's tax forms after someone dies.

How and where to renew the license registration for your vehicles

It's amazing. Usually just one person will take care of this yearly task and the other person may be clueless.

Talking about these things will not cause sudden disease. Writing a will is not going to hasten your death. Making your desires known to loved ones if you should become brain dead is not going to cause you to be hit by a train.

What **will** happen, is that your loved ones will be protected from feeling like a train has hit **them** if something unexpected happens to **you**. Doesn't the love you share make you to want to spare each other from added pain and trauma when faced with horrendous decisions at a time of crisis?

Both parties should have a working knowledge of bill paying, *location of important papers*, how to shut off the gas, water, and electricity, how to operate the generator (write these steps down), how to start the lawn mower and use it, how to do the laundry, and how to cook a meal.

Hopefully, "The Conversation" should happen years in advance. Once discussed, the topics should be revisited and updated with all involved as life situations change.

Take-Aways from Chapter 2:

- Part of the bedrock of caregiver survival is preparation

- Having "The Conversation" is based upon your mutual, supportive love
- Don't delay. Use the talking points in this chapter to get started.

3

DURING THE CAREGIVING TIME

This is where the rubber meets the road. It may be a very short period or one lasting years. My period of active, hospice-level caregiving lasted two years. I felt like I was going through the Biblical "Refiner's Fire"—being hardened, purified; shedding all that was not necessary; getting a clearer understanding of the everlasting quality of love—and coming out of that fire a changed person ... and all for the better.

I learned to live with grace. I lived because of grace. I became more graceful.

I also learned to walk on water.

Returning to Biblical analogies, I often felt like I was being asked to do the emotionally, mentally, and physically impossible. The equivalent of walking on water.

In the Bible story of Jesus walking on the water toward the disciples who were on a boat during a storm, Peter is bid by Jesus to get out of the boat to walk toward him. Peter starts stepping out and walking on the water but when he takes his eyes off of Jesus (his goal and source of strength) he starts to take in the sights and sounds of the storm about him. He flounders and falls into the waves, needing rescue.

As caregivers, we are called to keep our eyes on the love that drives us forward and keeps us afloat. If you are not a person of faith, keep your eyes on the bigger picture and beauty of your mutual love. As a believer, I kept my eyes on God; if I got distracted from my source of strength—and I sometimes did—then I would flounder in the storm of my very complex role as caregiver to my dying husband.

Walking on water is an imperfect practice. Using and seeking every resource available to you will help you gain the perspective you need to once again return your focus to seeing just the love. The wind and waves will not drown you with such a focus.

Seeking help

The time of caregiving is the time to call in the troops. You may be so used to putting other's needs first, but now it is supremely important to recognize your own. Remember, as the caregiver, if you collapse into a puddle or completely lose your own health, the whole system breaks down. Not only could *you* face a change of life and need a facility to rehab in, but your loved one will, too, because you won't be there!

This is a time of actively reaching out to others. You may be thinking that it's time for others to reach out to you, but do you know what it is like on the sidelines? People are generally clueless as to your needs. They don't know how to help you because they don't know what you need.

"Call me if you need anything," is usually the beginning and the end of helping efforts. Though offered in earnest, people don't know if you need a meal, or just want to be left alone. Trust me. You do not want to be left alone.

Being needy was definitely a new role for me. I sometimes felt a little awkward asking for help, but I realized I just had to keep myself going—and without help—that was not going to happen.

Once your circle of friends gets some experience helping you, they will have a better idea of what you need. They will understand when and how to reach out to you.

Maybe you don't know what you need? I've been there, too. That's probably when you need to reach out to others the most—when you are too numb to know that you need anything.

Throughout my caregiving, I would often call others just for a chat; to hear another voice; to be talked off an emotional ledge; to ask them over for a visit, or to make arrangements to meet for a meal.

My faith deepened dramatically during those two years of intense caregiving. I discovered, the more I gave our situation over to God, the more I saw His hand leading, guiding, directing, and sending help our way.

I also became so hyper-vigilant to every change in my husband's condition, I felt like an over-wound clock spring. Relaxing became almost impossible at times. Getting meaningful time off was an essential lifeline.

In order to maintain a healthy, restful state as a caregiver, having clear conversations with the patient about their care and your needs is very helpful. You may never get a "blessing" from the patient to be out of the house, but the reality of your need does not change just because they expect you at their beck-and-call 24/7. You must press on with weekly errands, time off for lunch with friends, and favorite activities that feed your soul.

Activities for you

Time away from caregiving is vital for survival. While my heart ached that my husband's world had shrunk to the size of his bed and room, I began to realize my world had shrunk as well. An endless horizon of being house bound with caregiving duties is a recipe for terrible mind games and madness.

Ways of getting help at home are discussed in the companion book to this: *Toolkit for Caregivers*. Trying to soldier through every monumental task of caregiving alone is not healthy. Becoming a martyr caregiver is pointless and totally unnecessary. Use the resources I shared in *Toolkit for Caregivers* to create a network of help for you and your loved one/patient.

Of course, leaving the house is a pleasure and yet, another opportunity for those conflicting feelings of guilt, as well. I simply was not prepared for so many random feelings of guilt that plagued me.

I could go out—he couldn't. I used to have a companion when going out in the world—now I didn't.

Errands had to be done. Groceries bought. Upon returning to the house, I would give my husband a full report of accomplishments and goodies procured for the coming meals. I handled outings that way because he was not resentful and enjoyed hearing about the outside world. Then I would do an activity with him. (Activities for the patient will be discussed next).

Glowing descriptions of the world outside of the patient's four walls could unintentionally create hurt feelings. Such sharing deserves discretion and thoughtfulness.

I quickly learned the importance of exercise and over-all body movement during my scheduled departures from the house. Even though I was a fully participating caregiver in all of my husband's needs, I still needed another type of movement. Getting enough exercise was a constant challenge and became a growing requirement for me.

While just getting out of the house, leaving all of the pressures behind, and sinking into a comfortable chair at a coffee shop or library may beckon and seem justified, some of your free time must include exercise—preferably with others because the social aspect is vital to survival.

Whether you ride a bike, go to group classes at the gym or YMCA, jog, hike, play tennis or basketball ... the endorphin release that comes with exercise is key to not only physical strength, but also mental and emotional resilience. Once a week is bare minimum; twice or more would be optimal. That's why it's so important to secure relief help for yourself throughout the week.

There's also exercise at home. I devote an entire chapter to easy and effective home exercises in my first book, *Toolkit for Wellness*. There's so much more than solitary jumping jacks and push-ups. Check out the whole range of possibilities you can do even while cooking in the kitchen!

At least twice a month, get together with a friend or two for a meal out. The best time in my husband's schedule for me to be gone was after his morning routine and breakfast. That meant my outings were usually from 10-2 pm while he napped and then ate lunch. So, as I went about my errands, eating a bite with friends was easy to arrange.

Having a friend over once a week for Happy Hour was an emotional life saver for me. Early on, we took the party to my husband's bedside where we shared beverages and a snack—and a lot of laughs. Later, when he was mostly sleeping, my friends and I would retire to the living room for a visit. Sometimes these visits extended into sharing dinner as well. This goes a long way to lifting everyone's spirits.

For the first year, adult coloring books were an integral part to centering my mind, calming my spirits, and offering a doable creative outlet. I could do this while my husband napped. Even just five minutes of coloring before I went to bed worked wonders to relax me. The thing about coloring is that the process is so absorbing, you do not think about anything else. Applying color to the page requires attention and concentration to the point that the cares of the day simply float away. Total magic. Try it.

I think I worked though my personal demons just coloring that first year. There were demons of self-pity, resentment, sorrow, and regret of what-would-not-be that needed to be viewed with some perspective. Coloring helped me do that, indirectly and subconsciously. Cheap therapy.

You're going to need it or something else you enjoy like it. One way or another, there are emotions that need to be processed. Becoming a caregiver will send you lots of emotions, indeed. A bucketful. Emotions that may blind-side you.

A doctor advised me early on that resentment would plague me if I wasn't careful in getting enough free time away. He had seen caregiving spouses become bitter from deep resentments. This was golden advice. While I did have mostly adequate outings, there was an element of resentment I had to process.

Whatever emotions you are feeling, it's normal. Normal! If you are having trouble processing all of it, that's normal, too. Get help. Friends. Pastors, Social Workers from your Home Health and Hospice agency, your doctor, a licensed therapist, or a group of caregivers. Reach out for help. It's a confusing time and a difficult time. Whatever you are feeling is legitimate and can be addressed. Get help.

Keep your passions alive. Garden club? Choir practice? Duck hunting? Time in the shop for wood working? Do not neglect your passions. Schedule time to regularly maintain your personal interests. I know you are a caregiver and every moment counts with your loved one, but short of staying there for the last breaths, life must go on. Your loved one—in their right mind—would not want you to fall off a cliff in despair.

Honor that. Live. As best you can.

Activities for your loved one/patient

Activities that cheer your loved one will also cheer you. It's a win-win.

Whether you are holding hands watching a favorite TV show or you are listening to some golden oldies you once enjoyed, activities do not have to be elaborate.

Music is particularly enjoyable to people and speaks to deep memories and happiness. The sense of sound lingers when other senses have gone and even when the patient is in an altered state.

A growing portion of our society is learning to live with, and support others, with severe dementia or Alzheimer's disease. Where your loved one is on the spectrum of dementia's severity will change over time and require evolving, adaptable approaches for patient involvement and connection.

Families dealing with dementia, especially, need a particular kind of support for their unique circumstances and stresses. I highly recommend asking the patient's doctor for local resources of support groups for caregivers. Those groups offer caregivers a connectivity, a chance to vent, a chance to hear about successful approaches, and provide more resources for them and their loved one/patient.

For all patients and their families, sticking to as normal a routine as possible is important. Keep your loved one/patient connected to family activities. If they are confined to a single room, bring the family meals to their room. They should never be left alone to eat. If the whole family cannot squeeze into the patient area, at least one other person should be eating with them from a plate balanced in their lap, if needed.

Love is inclusion. Whenever possible, include your loved one.

If your loved one can read, supplying them with a stream of reading materials is not hard, but maybe holding up a book and reading it are not on their radar. Audio books and playing devices are available from most libraries.

I can't count the number of books I read out loud to my husband. From animal stories, historical novels, mysteries, humor, philosophy, to romances. You name it. We read it. One of our favorite times to read was in the late afternoon before dinner. We shared a beverage and perhaps some pretzels and I would read. It was such an enjoyable experience that we both hated stopping so I could fix dinner. He would watch the news or take another snooze while I was in the kitchen.

One of our supplemental caregivers loved to read aloud to my husband. They kept their own set of reading materials exclusive to when she stayed with him. One night she was inspired to bring a hymnal and she sang to him while I was gone. He was able to sing along to the familiar tunes if he wanted.

Reviewing pictures with your loved one may be a memorable activity, as well—if their condition allows. Remember, advanced

Alzheimer's and dementia patients can get confused and agitated while looking at pictures of people they do not recognize.

We went through every photo album in the house, talking about each picture, laughing, remembering, and enjoying watching our family grow up again. We reviewed one album every day or so until they were all covered. Our love, once again, was strengthened during this time of sharing and reminiscing.

Cell phone pictures are easily revisited. If you have another, larger device such as an iPad or computer, viewing the screen will be easier and multiple people can see at the same time. Don't forget to share the latest Facebook feed of cute animal videos.

If your loved one can still safely do their favorite crafts, by all means supply them with the materials to do so. I recently read an article about an elderly bed-fast gentleman who occupies most of his free time by knitting caps for cancer patients and the homeless! He uses a circular device available at craft stores on which you "knit" without knitting needles. Not only was he creatively occupied but he was still a contributing member of society.

Passive, visual activities do not have to be limited to watching TV. Consider the environment in which your loved one lives. Are there beautiful pictures to look at? Are there seasonal holiday decorations? Is there a bird feeder outside the window? This topic is thoroughly discussed in *Toolkit for Caregivers*, along with different ideas that will bring life and activity to your loved one.

Having that heart-to-heart conversation

This conversation should probably not be a singular event. If you have the time, revisiting this topic is beautiful, necessary, therapeutic for all involved—yet sad, and terribly bittersweet. You will both find all the conflicting emotions of grieving right there in your mutual laps. Grab a Kleenex.

This is where you acknowledge the meaning of your deep love and your appreciation. Share with him/her how your mutual loving consideration for each other has made your life journey together such a pleasure. That, as painful as the thought is, life without them—whenever that may happen—will be made so much more tolerable because of your preparations.

Reassure them your love will endure for the ages—it is timeless. They will want to know that you are going to carry on. Of course, your heart will be broken and aching, but promise them that you will embrace life as best you can without them—and mean it.

Snippets and variations of this conversation should not be reserved to the last moments of life. I hope you are expressing love and appreciation for each other every day. Time is so short and totally unpredictable. Never wait to tell or show someone you love them.

More tasks to check off during the caregiving process

During this time, the caregiver needs to do a bit more pre-planning for the eventual end. Take this time to do a rough draft of your loved one's obituary. Know where to locate family pictures: saved on computer, phone, CDs, photo albums, etc.

Get the funeral arrangements started, if not done previously. This is where pre-planning is such a blessing.

———

Take-Aways from Chapter 3:

- You are in the WORK of caregiving, and you need help
- There are activities you can do to cope with, and lessen, your stress levels
- There must be time for you—schedule it!
- There are activities for your loved one/patient as well
- Tell them over and over of your love
- There's more pre-planning to do
- Get help when needed
- Help is always needed

4

A TIME OF TRANSITION

Many patients in their final days have a period of transition. When the end is truly near, there comes a time when they seem to hover between earth and heaven.

Hopefully, you've prepared him/her, and yourself, for this time by reinforcing the love you share and your appreciation for them; how much you are going to miss them and that you will always hold them in your heart; that because of your mutual loving foresight, you will be OK; and you will not crawl into a hole and waste away —that you will live the best you can without them there by your side.

This is the time to call in close family and friends for closure. My husband, ever the one to equip others for success in life, had thought of a word of wisdom for our daughter just prior to transition—she eagerly leaned in to receive his thought but he forgot it. He concluded that she, "probably already had things all figured out," which was the ultimate blessing, really.

There is no crystal ball as to timing. It's unique to each person. The average time for this final change can take up to 8-10 days. Even in this limbo period, when medications may be administered to ease their discomfort—continue with words of comfort and love. They can hear you, sense your touch, and your presence.

This is a time when the primary caregiver does not—in their heart —ever want to leave the bedside of their loved one. It's a tough call whether to leave the house or not. There's always the concern about wanting to be there for the end—but the end may be days away. Each situation is unique. That kind of high, poignant, emotional drama can leave you exhausted. It may be advisable to call in a relief caregiver so you can at least briefly get a breath of fresh air or a quick meal.

Permission

It sounds strange, but many people in transition seem to hang on for some reason—and there may well be a reason. Perhaps everyone they want is not yet around them. Maybe they need to hear a word of forgiveness—or a withheld word of love.

Or ... a withheld word of permission. Yes. Permission to pass—to let go—to follow the light—to join others in heaven—whatever you believe.

After days of hovering in transition, when all of our family was surrounding his bed, my husband briefly opened his eyes for the last time to see us. We reassured him we were all together to support each other. We loved him. It was okay. We were there.

He returned to his slumbering state. We continued to hold his hand, kiss his forehead, and administered medicine to keep him comfortable. Hours later, he passed.

The last breath

Many of us may hold visions of being there for someone's last breath. Families move heaven and earth to hold round-the-clock vigils to assure their loved one that they are not alone.

Some patients, however, seem to hang on until that very moment when people briefly exit their room. It seems they want to depart in private. They want to do their final business on their own; they want to spare their loved ones from the pain—who knows—but it often happens.

If you miss their final moments or if you are there holding their hands, I hope you have done the work of surrounding your loved one and yourself with enough love to float you through the next few days.

Look around. You are standing on holy ground that you have filled with Love.

And Love is a beautiful thing.

———

Take-Aways from Chapter 4:

- Transition is a special, even sacred time
- Your loved one can still absorb your sounds and touches
- Use this time to reaffirm your love and gratitude
- Assure your loved one life will be hard without them, but your love will always remain
- Give them permission to pass
- Their passing may occur even in your briefest absence; that's okay

- As long as you are all surrounded with Love, it's all good

5

AFTER

Even with loving consideration, pre-planning, and preparation, you have just experienced a life-changing loss.

A flood of emotions will wash over you and everyone else present. Invariably, you will try to put what you all have experienced in perspective: "He's in a better place now," "At least she is no longer in pain," "He'll get to see his parents now," and the like.

But you are grieving your loss, regardless.

It's okay.

Years ago, during one of those pre-planning conversations, we had both decided on cremation. My husband was pleased with the pottery urn I had purchased for his and my use. Right after he died, however, our children and I realized that, once his body was taken away by the funeral home, we would never see him again. Because of that, we held our own private late night family wake in the quiet and comfort of our own home.

For several hours, we rotated in an out of his room, letting the reality of it all sink in and to console one another. At one point, we raised a glass around him, toasting both, to him and to his love. At the last, we shared a bowl of his favorite ice cream around his bed.

Finally, we called the funeral home and my dear husband's earthly remains were taken away.

This is when, like us, you will be taking the first shaky steps into a world without your loved one in it.

Yet they **are** in it. They are inside of you. Love lives here **still**. As you cry into their pillow, still breathing in their scent, they are still around you and—moreover—they are in your heart, too. The room where they lived still holds a presence of love ... you can feel it.

Funeral preparations should be pre-arranged, but at least one visit to the funeral home may be needed to finalize arrangements. At this time, the obituary needs to be polished and finalized from your initial rough draft. The funeral home will take care of submitting it to the newspaper.

We selected to have the funeral home prepare a memorial slide show from pictures we provided. Actually looking at years of family history and our family's happiness proved to be quite healing. We were beginning to appreciate my husband's legacy from a new vantage point. We were walking through one of the initial tasks that would take us through the first few days without him.

One foot in front of the other.

Breathe. Remember to breathe.

After the necessary tasks related to the funeral are complete, there come more tasks. These tasks helped take me by the hand and guide me through the initial days and weeks following my husband's death. There's hardly time to grieve—there's still a lot of stuff to do.

————

Take-Aways from Chapter 5:

- Your loved one's presence is gone; your arms are empty, yet your heart is both full and broken
- In the course of duties, tasks, and responsibilities, you *will* successfully walk through the next hours and days
- Breathe
- The loving preparedness you have done will pay off big time in the coming weeks
- Hang on to love
- Let others take your hand and lead you

6

GRIEF

As mentioned earlier, we caregivers share a particular brand of grief. We knew the end was coming. We were there for every downhill step. We already grieved for what would no longer be. We were haunted daily with the question of when *it* would happen, forever changing our world. We may have—guiltily—longed for the whole thing to be over—and then cried to make things last. What a crooked road we have walked.

Have we done all of our grieving? No. Real grieving will come.

As mentioned earlier, there hardly seems to be time enough to tackle our emotions because the business side of dying quickly takes center stage. But grief does trickle through between—and even during—the related chores we must go through. Sometimes, it will come unexpectedly when you're driving down the street—a wave of tears will hit you. Or watching his/her favorite show for the first time without them.

For me, writing thank you notes was Kleenex time. I tried to do several personal thank you notes every few days. They were written to those who gave flowers, showed special kindnesses, and donated memorial gifts. Seeing this flood of generosity and love from others just got to me. I was so very grateful and humbled.

Sucker-punch grief

It started out like a normal Tuesday. The business side of dying had been completed and I was establishing a new routine.

Tuesday mornings are highlighted by aerobics class at the gym. I was looking forward, as always, to this socially and physically stimulating time with an amazing instructor who puts a smile on our lips and sweat on our brows.

Doorbell rings. A man introduces himself as the tree trimmer who will be cutting down the neighbor's tree right next to our property. The tree is actually so big, it is pushing on the fence separating our properties. Would it be alright to let some branches fall on our open land and maybe drive their truck on it?

Well, okay. Sure. We had long wished for that pine tree to come down intentionally in a tree-trimming process rather than in a storm.

There's an hour before I needed to leave for aerobics class—better take a before picture. Share it with our kids who witnessed this tree grow from a sapling to the thirty-foot giant it now is. I take a picture. Click.

Sipping my coffee on the back porch, I never saw it coming.

Click. A before picture. First limb coming down. Click. Gee, the birds are going to miss this tree. Sitting on the top branches they view the whole neighborhood expanse. Squirrels race up and down its trunk and branches, feasting on the pine cone seeds.

More pictures are taken: click, click, click. Branches are being extracted one by one with precision care by the project master strapped to the trunk. Assistants on the ground below guide the felled branches with ropes.

Why am I suddenly feeling so sad? The lower branches clutter the ground, but where they came from is obscured by a tree of our own. No one would know the tree was slated to come down.

Wait! That next branch seems to have a squirrel's nest in it. Hope it's an old nest or else somebody's going to not have a home tonight.

Then the symbolic parallels hit. BAM! This is like watching my husband slowly die. This is terrible. I don't want to have this tree die; I don't want to see this! But somehow, I am riveted to the scene. Our whole family watched this tree grow up. Part of me is tied to this tree. I look at it countless times a day. It's a part of our visual and mental environment—our world.

This tree is going down—and rightfully so—and there's nothing I can do to stop it.

As I prepare a second cup of coffee, continuing my vigil and watching through the kitchen window, the gasping, tear-filled cries begin. Fists pound the counter top to no avail. The tree is being picked apart. My husband died cell by cell over two years (his own words). I had watched. I am watching again. This is tearing me apart.

Returning to the porch, I continue to witness this methodical death scene. Click. Click. Click.

Clearly this tree is losing its SELF. Still a tree, but greatly diminished. Sometimes I missed the change while glancing away.

Click.

Where did *that* branch go?

Other times, I watched as a now useless limb dangles by the rope and is guided to the ground.

Click.

Is the master trimmer going to lop off the tree top now, or will more branches yet be removed?

Click.

Click.

Looks like more will be removed before the final cut is made.

The cicadas have been buzzing all morning during this death scene. Humming birds come to the feeder. Dragon flies fill the air, doing their lovely job of cleaning the air of smaller flying insects. Thank you dragon flies! Life is going on all around. Birds glide in the air currents.

The master trimmer studies his work. Nothing is happening without his thoughtful skill and practiced insight.

I am reminded of my own Master. I always knew He was in control. The days or moments when I was most frustrated, overwhelmed, or anxious, were the days I did not keep my eyes focused on Him. Putting it ALL into His hands is what got me through—and is what is getting me through—this whole process.

Finally, it looks like the last cut is coming.

There. Click.

Not there. Click.

It's over. Nothing left to do but remove the trunk. I feel the ground shake as the trunk is dismantled and ultimately felled.

Boom. Boom. BOOM!

Done.

Death.

Burial or cremation.

The skyline is devoid of this once lovely tree.

This morning's trembling-lipped sobbing has abated for now. I will go out to do the delayed errands. Exercise will have to wait for Thursday.

Getting through the firsts

That first year will be full of emotional land mines. It will be a series of firsts. First birthday, anniversary, Thanksgiving—all through the year. Every holiday, every land mark—without your loved one.

For me, leaving town for many of these events seemed the best. After the business side of dying was concluded, I enjoyed reconnecting with friends and family. In fact, all major holidays have been spent out of town this first year.

I discussed this with our Hospice social worker. Was leaving town a form of escapism and denial? She said, just being aware and asking that, showed it was probably a good thing and not denial. There were still tearful moments, sure; but being alone in the house for holidays is probably not the best thing.

Coming home from trips can be a challenge though. I was coming home to the new reality and it hit me every time—but to lesser and lesser degrees as the number of trips expanded. Just a part of the grief journey, I guess.

Part of living with grief is getting enough *new* life to spring up on our life canvas. At first, our canvas is nothing but a picture of sorrow. Ever so gradually, that part of the picture either gets smaller or our canvas actually grows to include new life around the sadness.

I think it's the process of growth. My progress has included personal growth projects. My canvas of life is getting BIGGER.

I recall a memorial in the local park sponsored by our funeral home. We were there to remember our loved ones, share a pleasant meal in the open air, hear about grief counseling opportunities, share wisdom gained through grief, and to set loose a memorial balloon containing our loving wishes to the departed.

The lady across the table from me seemed to be so deeply sad, so deeply discouraged. Her husband had been gone longer than mine. I was reminded that each of us grieves in a unique way—there's no time schedule and we are not to judge.

I just know that, for myself, each new activity mostly brings me joy because I am able to seek the joy in everything. There's always that zinger that I am not doing this new activity with my husband, but—overall—I aim to achieve a sense of growth and enrichment in all that I do.

I strive to still see, hear, experience, and appreciate the life around me. I listen for the birds and cicadas. I see the hummers and dragon flies. Life is all around. I am in this life. My love and memories live in my heart and mind.

Personal Growth Opportunities

No longer being a caregiver—forgive me here—*freed* me to travel to distant family and friends. We used to do a bit of traveling together, a lot—in fact—over the years; but the last few years had seen us tied to home. Still balancing the ever present mélange of joy-guilt-regret, I have taken several trips to catch up with loved ones.

The joy part is getting bigger with each trip. I had promised my husband I would live a full life, write books, and stay fiscally responsible. I am fulfilling my promises.

Being without him is hard. I want to turn to him and make a comment about what I just saw or heard. The sharing component is deeply missed.

Lately, I am sometimes feeling sad at just being solo without a male partner. Maybe that's progress. I also promised to not turn away from dating and marrying someone else.

Steps. Baby steps.

Staying engaged with your local commitments is so important. Keep involved with your poker or bridge group. Keep active in your memberships with the book club, the men's prayer group, ladies groups, choirs, hunting club, etc.

Then, there comes a time to s-t-r-e-t-c-h. You may not feel like it, but join in on some new activities so that the view around you is new and not reminiscent of your loved one. So often we feel sad thinking about how we used to do this or that together. By doing something totally new, you are putting a memory stamp on an activity that's just yours.

Volunteer at the hospital, answer the phone at church, teach others to read, go to lectures at the local college, or volunteer as an usher at the community theater. The possibilities are endless.

I've always heard that, those who lose spouses, should not make major changes that first year. Certainly, there are many mitigating factors that would modify that adage—but you *can* change the focus and environment of your activities.

Follow a passion that has not yet been developed. Have you always been a camera bug? Take some classes in photography. Spread your wings.

Learn. Grow.

A friend of mine who was a former nurse and teacher decided to follow her photography passion after her husband died. In addition to becoming an award-winning nature photographer, she is a member of photography clubs, goes to shows and conventions, and travels with groups and by herself to take pictures outdoors.

Her transformation from early widowhood to present day nature photographer has been spectacular. Her journey is not aimed at fame and fortune. Her journey is aimed at self-fulfillment. There's no telling what someone can accomplish with a seed of curiosity and some consistent effort.

If you find yourself not regularly participating in the life around you, that is a cry for help. If you are lacking any motivation to get out of bed or take care of yourself, those who depend on you, or your surroundings, then you are among those who need help. Your doctor should be the first call. There are medications that can help you through that tough hump of depression while you possibly join a group for grief counseling.

Take-Aways from Chapter 6:

- Caregivers experience anticipatory grief in addition to normal grief
- Grief is unpredictable—sometimes you just seem to go along for the ride
- We are still living and should be participating in this life on earth
- Explore the endless world of personal growth
- There are resources readily available to help you through debilitating grief
- Ask for help

7

THE BUSINESS SIDE OF DYING

If you have prepared with thorough, loving consideration, you will love your dearly departed even more as you go about the business side of dying, because you will know exactly where everything is and what you need to do.

Death Certificates

I was issued three with the funeral arrangement package, and I purchased three more. The funeral home handled all of this. I found that our bank and our credit union were happy to just photocopy an original. The electric company and the cable provider also were satisfied in making photocopies. The annuities and investment companies all required an original (raised seal) death certificate.

It's also a good idea to get an official statement from the funeral home that the funeral expenses have been paid in full. The Clerk of Court's office needed to see that paper and make a copy.

What needs to be accomplished is to notify governmental, financial and legal institutions of your loved one's death and to get all accounts switched over to your name, closed out, or benefits collected.

These business affairs are addressed **after** the funeral. Give yourself a few days. When you do get the official death certificates from the funeral home, **then** you may begin your check list.

Unofficial Check List for the Business Side of Dying

County Clerk of Court—This should be your first stop.

In my state, because we had done our homework with a Last Will and Testament in place, joint accounts and house titles with Right of Survivorship, I did not have to open an estate on my husband's behalf.

Having said that, even though we jointly owned our cars, there was no Right of Survivorship duly noted on the title. Therefore, the Clerk of Court took the blue book value of both cars and subtracted that sum from the $60,000 allowable property value*. I was able to get the car titles in my name after a trip to the titling agency. If sometime down the road I find some real property I did not know about, it can come off of the remaining balance from that original $60,000 without having to open an estate.

*Our county offers this amount of property that does not require opening an estate. Your own county will have different guidelines.

If you do have to open an estate, the Clerk of Court will help you establish in what county the estate will be opened.

- The estate will be opened in the county of permanent personal residence of the deceased. Even if land is owned in other counties, the owner's personal residence is the determining factor.

- NOTE to people who live on their boat or in an RV with no permanent personal residence. Opening an estate could be problematic due to lack of a permanent residence. Usually, a P.O. Box is not a qualifying address. Those enjoying the good life on the road or in the waters fulltime should work with their attorney in establishing a workable permanent address for estate purposes.

Your Clerk of Court will guide you through each step of opening an estate.

Your subsequent business stops should include:

- Banks, savings accounts
- Credit Unions
- Credit cards
- Social Security—there's a possible Social Security Death Benefit for which you may qualify
- Veteran's Administration, if applicable
- County Tax Office, if you pay county taxes on real property
- Cell phone
- Cable, satellite, internet companies
- Telephone
- Electric company
- Gas company
- Water company
- Loan companies—including school loans
- House and property insurance companies (often overlooked by survivors)
- Annuities

- Life insurance
- Stocks and investments
- IRAs and Roth accounts
- If the deceased was enrolled in a private school or institution of higher learning, check for possible refund of unused paid fees

If you have a legal advisor, check with them if you have any questions. The originals of our Medical and Legal Power of Attorney and Last Will and Testament were on file at our attorney's office. The Clerk of Court needed the original Last Will and Testament for my husband to keep on file, and our county, as a courtesy, offered to keep mine in a secured, confidential file as well.

More Tasks to Do

One of the best condolence gifts came in a sympathy card which contained several pages of pretty stamps for me to use on the thank you notes. I will never forget that gift.

Speaking of thank you notes, pace yourself in completing them. People do not expect you to acknowledge a sympathy card but outright gifts of money, memorials, food, and other kindnesses should be addressed. Just doing these simple tasks will be healing. Keep a box of Kleenex nearby as tears will flow. That's normal and appropriate.

Most funeral homes will supply the bereaved with complimentary generic thank you notes and will even mail them free of charge when you drop them back off after completion. We decided, however, to find a pack of more personal note cards on our own. Using my friend's stamp gift, I was all set to write thank you notes and mail them myself.

―――――

Take-Aways from Chapter 7:

- Walking through the business of dying will actually help you keep putting one foot in front of the other.
- Even with perfect preparedness, there are places to contact about your loved one's passing
- "Thank you" note writing is a part of the healing and grieving process. Embrace it.

8

LEARNING TO SEE THE WORLD WITH A NEW FOCUS

You have accomplished quite a lot. You have loved. You have been loved. That's a "Wow!" on any scale.

But life has clearly changed.

You have come through your caregiving role and are no longer the same person. Chances are, you are battle worn and suffer from deep fatigue. You feel more than a little emotionally and physically exhausted or beat up.

A part of you feels relief—but then the feelings of guilt rush in at even thinking such things. It's true, though. Mixed thoughts and emotions continue to flood you. It's perfectly okay to embrace that relief, and it's natural to have that spoiler pang of guilt. Just know that these jumbled emotions are normal when you experience things such as:

- The first time you leave the house without arranging someone to stay with your loved one in your absence.
- The first time you enjoy an uninterrupted meal.

- The first time you get only yourself ready for bed and not your loved one first.

The time will come, however, when you **will** enjoy a beautiful day for what it is. A beautiful day with you in it.

Not a beautiful day without your loved one but just a beautiful day with you in it.

Look around. What else is beautiful? Where can you create more beauty?

Walk toward that. Live that.

And yet, there's that love. It still lives but in a different way—deep within the heart. I still find comfort sitting in a chair we moved to the space my husband's bed occupied. I love to read in that spot. I had read countless books out loud in that room. Reading by myself in that spot feels right because now I am in some of the physical space he once occupied, and I find peace there.

Seek out and appreciate the bright spots.

Reframe your focus to concentrate not on what *isn't* there, but the goodness that *is* there.

Survival Tip

Help Yourself.

One day nearly three months into widowhood, I found myself flopping down on the bed for yet another rest. This was more than jet lag from my recent 28-day vacation of rest and relaxation with family and friends. I had taken a 4-hour nap earlier to satisfy the jet lag. This smacked of depression.

Was I going to lie here forever? Felt like it.

The words, "help yourself," rang out in my mind.

I knew how to fix this—help myself. Get my butt off the bed and go out to the waterfront park for a walk. No one was going to do it for me. Only I could help myself. If I wanted to feel better, I had to do something about it. Get out. Move around. See what was happening in my town. Breathe some fresh air.

So I did.

With the same enthusiasm one would have while tying shoelaces, I sort of robotically got up, combed my hair, got my bag and keys, and drove to the park.

Turned out to be a lovely evening; still a warm and humid August evening but with a refreshing breeze. There were kids running around kicking balls, swinging on swings. Folks walking their dogs. Others out for the evening, strolled by the river. Music was floating in the air from outdoor restaurants. Beautiful clouds mounded up like whipped cream, and there were early signs of a gorgeous sunset.

One foot in front of the other.

Walk.

Breathe.

Greet strangers with a sincere smile.

I took a memory shot of the fantastic sky, then put the cell phone away and absorbed the present moments.

That one effort of helping myself—albeit reluctantly—changed my whole outlook.

I am reminded that grief is a solo journey.

Ultimately, I have to help myself.

———

Take-Aways from Chapter 8:

- You have loved and you have been loved back. That is a wonderful thing.
- Refocus on what is, not what is no longer
- Living our lives today does not dishonor those who no longer live here with us.
- The love never dies; and should become that glowing ember in our hearts that warms and comforts us.
- Continue to grow, to reach out to others.
- Appreciate today with you in it.

CONCLUSION

There is no conclusion to grief.

But because of **loving preparedness**, you can enter into, and emerge from, a caregiving role much stronger, less damaged, and more resilient.

Have you heard others offer advice to, "embrace the pain/grief"? I never really understood that until the second year of my caregiving ministrations. Because I had no book like this one to read, it took me a year to get my head screwed on straight. We knew—sort of— that we'd be in this for a long haul.

That second year, I had a healthier perspective and adequate help. One day, after reading a description of a book about selecting a *word for the year*, a word came to my mind—out of the blue. Embrace.

I needed to embrace every aspect of my life. Embrace and lean into the love, the grief, the work of caregiving, the work of love, my dear husband, our situation, the day, and the ups and downs ... everything.

When I was truly embracing, I was not fighting, or resenting, or resisting. That's being a healthy caregiver.

Many books have dissected the grief process and techniques for coping. This tiny tome was not created to replace them. This is intended to be a nuts-and-bolts approach to a very complicated series of life events and preparations. Short and quick.

As a former caregiver and as a new widow, my attention span is short. I did not want to challenge yours while sharing this information. I have worked hard to not add fluff to this book—to just give everything to you straight.

Hopefully, this book will become the springboard you need to:

- Prepare for your caregiving duties way before you become a caregiver
- See you through the mental, emotional, and physical challenges of being a caregiver
- Provide an understanding about end-of-life needs
- Help you through the immediate issues in the business side of dying
- Get you through your early grief, and
- Help you discover possibilities for your continued life without your loved one at your side.

THANK YOU READERS

If you have been helped by reading this book and by using some of this information, please share *Toolkit for Caregivers/Love Lives Here, Toolkit for Caregiver Survival* with another person who is in need of help, support, and guidance. We caregivers have to stick together.

Requests for seminars, discounts for bulk purchases of this book, questions or comments may be sent to me at: deidre@toolkitsforhealth.com

Please check out my blogs at https://foodtalk4you.com and http://deidreedwards.com, where I address personal wellness, "one meal, one breath, one movement at a time."

May each of you come through the refiner's fire a new and better person.

May you be able to enjoy the sunshine on your face because *you* are in the day.

It will happen!

ACKNOWLEDGMENTS

Again, all glory goes to God who encouraged me to write this. I felt inspired—anointed even—as I fleshed out a bare bones outline of ideas on paper into a cohesive whole book in a week's time. A companion survivor's book to *Toolkit for Caregivers* just **had** to be written. My readers needed the rest of the story!

Deep thanks to Virgil, my beloved husband, now in heaven, who was instrumental in our mutual loving preparedness. While he handled the business side of our family life, he made sure to always include me in understanding how that aspect of our lives was run. I was never clueless. He was equally prepared to do my tasks should I have become disabled.

James and Serena, our two wonderful children, and I seek every opportunity to connect and support each other as our small family's dynamic changes. They applaud and support my writing and outreach projects in every way possible. Thank you both—we are cumulatively doing what Dad would have wanted us to do.

Thank you to those around me who remarked, "How did you know what all to do after your husband died?" Those remarks sealed the deal in making me want to complete this book. Each of us should not have to re-invent the wheel. While not an exhaustive list, my *Business Side of Dying* check list should certainly get you started and headed in the right direction.

Sheree Alderman, my editor, continues to supply laser-focused changes and ideas that help make my outreach in words so much more effective. We still talk each other off of the proverbial ledge from time to time. We still need that writers' retreat, girl.

Longtime friend, Betty Eliopulos, and her husband Eli Demas, have given me the soul-boosting support I needed so badly as a new widow. "Thank you" is inadequate to express my heartfelt gratitude to you both and to my whole circle of new friends in Roseville, California, as well. Betty, your serving as a beta reader and giving feedback was crucial in pushing me forward with this project.

Charlotte Fuller, from the Craven County Clerk of Courts Office, guided me through much of the business side of dying for my husband. She also assisted me in understanding the bigger picture of estate processes and some of the special concerns that often occur. Thank you so much!

RESOURCES

Here are some resources that would be helpful to all readers:

- https://foodtalk4you.com—my blog posts about mind/body/spirit wellness
- *Toolkit for Wellness—Master Your Health and Stress Response for Life*—Deidre Edwards
- *Reframe Your Viewpoints*—Virginia Ritterbusch
- *Out of the Maze*–Spencer Johnson, M.D.
- *The 18 Rules of Happiness*—Karl Moore
- *Choosing Happy*—Heidi Farrelly

ABOUT THE AUTHOR

Although Deidre Edwards first began as a nursing instructor, helping students in the healthcare industry—her latter efforts in writing and personal appearances have proven very successful as well—having focused both, students and readers, on navigating and succeeding in whatever tasks were before them.

While writing her second book, *Toolkit for Caregivers—Tips, Skills, and Wisdom to Maximize Your Time Together*, it became apparent that a supplemental book was needed to prepare her readers for "the rest of the story."

Fresh from living the early days of widowhood, Deidre has taken the topic of caregiving to its natural conclusion. What will happen when caregiving days are over? There's a whole new learning curve, and Deidre can't resist trying to help others through those next steps as painlessly as possible.

She discovered that successful navigation of those next steps was contingent upon skills practiced years before. Those skills were based upon loving consideration. She is hoping that readers may benefit from "The Conversation" talking points years in advance to becoming a caregiver.

She also understands that many may not have that time of preparation. Wherever her readers are in their life stages—young and healthy to the very old—there are many handy tools presented here to make any kind of caregiving journey smoother.

Deidre wants to remind her informed readers that she is sharing her experiences; she does not claim to be a licensed legal professional or medical adviser. All of her readers should contact their own legal and medical professionals for guidance specific to their own situations.

To contact Deidre, email her at deidre@toolkitsforhealth.com. She can help you with reduced prices for bulk purchases of her books and for group seminars as described on her business site: DeidreEdwards.com.

Made in the USA
Las Vegas, NV
08 September 2022

54906113R00115